Hafsa Tameez likes to consider herself a jack-of-all-trades and may have more grandiose dreams than she has time to pursue. She is an interior designer, a cultural heritage management expert, and a lifelong devotee of the anime world. She's not entirely convinced superpowers are not real and is immovably certain her cat is out to get her.

Dedicated to you who picked up this book, to all the socially anxious out there, and to the friends and family that keep us putting one step in front of another.

Hafsa Tameez

OF BUTTERFLIES AND COCOONS

Understanding the S.A.D. Mind

AUSTIN MACAULEY PUBLISHERS™
LONDON • CAMBRIDGE • NEW YORK • SHARJAH

Copyright © Hafsa Tameez (2021)

The right of Hafsa Tameez to be identified as author of this work has been asserted by the author in accordance with Federal Law No. (7) of UAE, Year 2002, Concerning Copyrights and Neighboring Rights.

All rights reserved. No part of this publication may be reproduced, stored in a retrieval system, or transmitted in any form or by any means; electronic, mechanical, photocopying, recording, or otherwise, without the prior permission of the publishers.

Any person who commits any unauthorized act in relation to this publication may be liable to legal prosecution and civil claims for damages.

Austin Macauley is committed to publishing works of quality and integrity. In this spirit, we are proud to offer this book to our readers; however, the story, the experiences, and the words are the author's alone.

The age category suitable for the books' contents has been classified and defined in accordance to the Age Classification System issued by the National Media Council.

ISBN – 9789948844266 – (Paperback)
ISBN – 9789948844259 – (E-Book)

Application Number: MC-10-01-1848697
Age Classification: 17+

Printer Name: iPrint Global Ltd
Printer Address: Witchford, England

First Published (2021)
AUSTIN MACAULEY PUBLISHERS FZE
Sharjah Publishing City
P.O Box [519201]
Sharjah, UAE
www.austinmacauley.ae
+971 655 95 202

The completion of this work would not have been possible without the unending support from my parents, my brother, and the indomitable Faryal Anjum, Gayathri Ravindran, and Revathy Ramakrishnan. Without all of their unrelenting encouragement to pursue this project – yes I need that many people to get off my tush and accomplish something worthwhile – I would not have been able to climb the mountain of putting my thoughts into words. And I certainly would not have been able to find the courage to put those words out there for someone else to read. I offer them my greatest debt of gratitude, a lifetime supply of coffee, and the rest of my life at their beck and call.

I would like to thank the laundry list of therapists who have tried in their own ways to keep me going. Well done, chaps. I'm still here.

I would also like to thank all the people I talk about in the pages to come, because without them I would not have arrived to where I am now. They made me who I am today and I do believe I am stronger for their contributions.

And lastly, I want to thank you. Yes, you. Thank you for trying to make life a happier experience, whether for yourself or for others around you. And for buying this book 'cause LOL I didn't think anyone would. You have fallen into my spider web. And now welcome to my world.

If this ever sees the light of day, then that means I succeeded.
And you can too.

A Word, If I May

If I may afford myself the opportunity to be honest for once in my life, I would admit that I don't know how to start. I know what I want to do, what I want this to accomplish. But to do that I must remember that which I wish I could forget: Myself.

Yes, starting is always the hardest.

Especially for people like me.

So perhaps I should start with a warning. Oh ye faint of heart, leave this tale of woe and misery whilst thou still can. This tale shall get graphic, this tale shall get violent, this tale shall get depressing.

This tale is very lonely.

Now that that is out of the way, let me bite the bullet and rip the band-aid off and jump in the deep end. I shall introduce myself.

When I started writing this, it was my last day of being 25. And, for the first time, I woke up happy.

That's a rare thing for me. I think I'm a happy person, but then again, I don't think I am.

You're going to learn a few things about me. One of them is that I don't make a lot of sense. I'm a jumble of contradictions. Someone once said that I was special. Yeah, I'm special all right. The special-est of all the special snowflakes.

It's OK; you'll get used to my brand of self-deprecating humor.

You see, there's something you must know about me: there's something wrong with me. My mom would deny it, and my doctor will try to bend my mind into thinking there's nothing 'wrong' per say. But the truth of the matter is, that's how I feel.

Wrong.

I live with a condition called social anxiety disorder. I have had it all my life.

Now before you put this down and shake your head going 'ah another self-proclaimed mentally ill martyr about to go on a self-pity trip' let me assure you, that's not what this is. Whatever *this* is.

Yes, you're right, I did grow up misunderstood by the people around me. For all our modernity and progress and whatnot, I firmly believe that we as a society do not understand what social anxiety is. We know the definition, we know what it means on paper half the time. But you don't know what life is like in my head. You can't know how my mind works and how it thinks and how it takes logic and shoves it out the window of a very high story building.

That's exactly why this, writing this, is important. 'Cause growing up *sucked*. And being the incorrigible bleeding heart that I am, I wouldn't wish my childhood upon anyone else. So here's to hoping this makes even a bit of difference for someone out there. Whether you're like me, or know someone like me, or maybe you're just trying to broaden your literary horizons; welcome. Welcome to me baring my heart – not in a kinky way – and hoping that my insight might make a difference to someone.

Part One: Anagnorisis

I am what you call your average raging lunatic. I wasn't always like this but I guess no one really is. You can argue nature versus nurture all day but we will still arrive at the same intriguing conclusion; I'm a lunatic *now*. Doesn't really matter how I got here. What matters is where I go from here. Deep, isn't it? Yeah, I have my moments.

I was born Hafsa Tameez. Actually it's Hafsa Tameez Ahmed Junejo, but since nobody can properly pronounce the last name I decided to stop at Tameez. Also 'cause Ahmed gets me in trouble at airports.

I'm Pakistani. In my passport at least. Not so much in my head or in my little unpatriotic heart.

Instead, and I am wildly aware of how cheesy this is going to sound, I like to think of myself as a global nomad. Yeah, I felt the cringe too.

I was two and a half when we moved to Sudan. And that's where my childhood begins.

I spent a lot of time wandering the neighborhood streets, befriending the stray cats and riding my little rainbow-colored bike with the training wheels, while my parents tried to find me a suitable school.

I loved school. At first. My mother helped me prepare and came to drop me off on my first day in the playgroup. She intended to stay in the school for a few hours to help me adjust but I guess I threw a wrench in her considerate plan. In a story my mother likes to tell, I apparently told her to get lost and that she was too old for school. And so she went home.

I turned out to be rather good at this school thing. I was quiet and well-behaved and the teachers loved me. Academia came easily to me too. I remember the day I first learned to read. The class was seated on the floor in a group while the teacher tried her best to teach us that when we see 'A' we read it as 'aah.' I remember only half-focusing on her lesson after 10 minutes of repetition and turning instead to the alphabet cards pasted on the wall. I focused on the first word and tried to read it. It was too hard, so I moved on to the second one. 'Bah,' 'aah,' 'nuh,' 'aah,' 'nuh,' 'aah.' I remember the elation of the moment when baahnuhaanuaah turned into 'banana.' The absolute glee! I turned to the teacher ecstatic, and waited patiently for everyone to stop talking so I could tell her 'Banana!'

That moment never came, and I wasn't confident enough to interrupt. A few days later I cornered her alone during painting time and led her to the letters on the wall again. "Fuh-oh-kss," I read. "Fox!"

I turned to her, utterly proud of myself for mastering a hard word with an x in it. The teacher's jaw dropped and she quickly had me try again. "Appleh," I read, followed by "umbrelela." Close enough for a three-year-old. English is dumb.

I was put in the advanced reading group by myself, a position I was proud to uphold throughout my academic career.

I remember being quite lonely as a child. So much so that when my parents announced that I might be getting a sibling, I fell in love with the idea. "I want a baby brother," I ordered my rather rueful parents. Luckily God decided to grant my wish and eight months later I was a proud, overprotective older sister to a little blue lizard I called my brother. Not a pet; my brother was born premature and for some reason he was deprived of oxygen and was born blue.

My brother, whom I proudly named Osama after my school bus driver 'cause I thought it was a cute name, was the absolute opposite of me. Where I was a quiet and gentle toddler, he was a raging ball of bare-bottomed hyper energy. And we got along swimmingly.

I remembered traveling a lot as a child. My father is an ophthalmologist, an eye surgeon. And he had the honor of working for an NGO that brought medical aid to underprivileged areas in rural Africa. He would leave for eye camps, where a team of doctors and technicians would spend days, or weeks, performing free eye surgery in some far away village.

I remember spending a lot of time in the office hi-lux pick-up. My favorite memory perhaps is driving through the desert after a gentle Saharan rain. The dunes were tranquil, the sky a painted canvas of yellows and blues and grays. The weather was a rare perfect and so we decided to stop for a bit.

I took this time to go exploring. I climbed the dunes, I proclaimed myself king of the sandy mountain. And then tumbled down the side only to climb up and do it all over again. At some point I decided to explore the back side of the dune. No one was watching me, all the men busy trying to make tea on a coal brazier, and so I took that as a sign to do whatever I want. When I went around the other side, I noticed something odd. The rain had washed some of the dunes' sides away and there, exposed to see was what looked to be the skeleton of a large fish, with a pointed nose, kind of like a swordfish. It was a magnificent sight. I couldn't resist the urge to reach out and touch it. As soon as I did, it crumbled to dust, melting away with the rest of the sand. I immediately recoiled, horrified, and scampered off to join the rest of the party as if nothing had happened. I don't even know if the memory is real, but the magnificence and mystery of the Saharan desert definitely left an impact on me for the rest of my life. Just don't tell an archaeologist that I may have accidentally destroyed a piece of evidence of life in the Sahara millions of years ago. Shhh.

By the time I hit seven years, I had to switch schools. The one that I got accepted to had a nationwide entrance exam that you had to pass. Apparently I got the second highest score in Sudan, but I have never been able to find evidence of that so maybe my parents just made that up to make me happy.

It was a huge school, and I learned to hate it. Ha, see? I *am* normal. There were simply too many people. I also learned kids could be really cruel and it was my first time being introduced to the universal concept of the 'bully.'

Luckily I didn't stay there long and after a year, we had to move back to Pakistan. Those were not happy times. Neither my brother nor I had grown up Pakistani. We couldn't speak the language and we were untrained in the never-ending list of complicated and often contradictory customs. What made it worse was that my father was constantly traveling back to Africa for his job, leaving my mother alone to care for us, the household, the finances, her job as a teacher, the car, and a laundry list of other chores including the actual laundry.

My brother and I were enrolled in the school my mother worked at. It was an entirely new atmosphere and I learned very quickly to resent the idea of school. I am fairly certain we were only allowed in because my brother and I spoke English, a fact that our principal made ample use of to publicize her institution. Often I was called in to her office to speak with prospective parents in English to show off the school's standard. Her biggest gambit was to sign me up for a debate competition and had me practice my speech for how brains were better than brawn in front of the whole school. The constant practice was a nightmare and I realized early on that I did not like crowds. I didn't like being in them, and I certainly didn't like being in front of them. My hands went cold and things would get very loud in my head.

On the day of the actual competition, I found out two horrible things. The competition was televised live in Pakistan. And the competition was for high schoolers. I was barely in the fifth grade! Surrounded by these tall, mature girls, I had never felt so ill-prepared or so inadequate. One after the other they got up to perform, each confident and bold and so sure of her points. And with each person, I sank further into my seat.

Finally, my name was called, and at first I couldn't move. Maybe if I refused to go up there, they wouldn't make me talk in front of the crowd. I wasn't so lucky. The girl next to me pushed me out of my seat and shoved me toward the stage. Shakily I got up the steps. The moderator asked me what my topic was and I whispered it so low he had to put his ear in front of my mouth to catch my words. He nodded, then gestured to the podium. But I was too short to reach the top and he had to pause amidst a giggle from the audience while they got me a stool to stand on. The moderator picked me up and deposited me on the stool at the podium, and I immediately blanked out. The crowd dissolved into a sea of featureless faces with large gaping eyes all focused on me. My legs were shaking so hard and I desperately needed to pee. I wanted to throw up and all I could focus on was the feeling that the ceiling of the great hall at the venue was spinning. I opened my mouth…

And was awoken by applause. Apparently I had won third place and this time the girl next to me did nothing to help me get back up on the stage to accept my award. Instead the moderator from earlier had to motion furiously for me to get my little butt up there.

Two things changed after that day. I became more subdued. Instead of boosting my confidence at so great an accomplishment, I felt humiliated somehow. I felt like I had robbed some girl of the prize; I mean I was only eleven, I didn't even deserve to be at the competition in the first place!

And second, the school turned on me. 'Teacher's pet' was my nickname and my fellow students were not as shy as I was about letting me know exactly what they thought of me. I apparently spoke Urdu with a funny accent. My English accent was just as ridiculous. I was fat and short. My hair looked stupid. My handwriting was hideous. I was ugly. I didn't have friends because I was dumb. The list grew every day.

Luckily I didn't have to stay there much longer and after I was done with primary school, I was moved to a public school for sixth grade. Public school offered me something I realized I was quick to grow too comfortable with: invisibility. My class section had upward of fifty students in it. And I disappeared into the crowd. This time I made sure to keep my head down and blend in. I didn't let anyone sign me up for speech competitions or drama shows or debates. I refrained from getting the first position in class and was happy being second. And I realized that I grew very lonely very quickly.

Around this time, while I was wrestling with the perks and drawbacks of anonymity, my father moved to Niger for a one-year contract, leaving us alone for the first time for so long a period. The initial plan was that he would come back after a year because they didn't want to interrupt my brother's and my education. Oh, how I longed for Africa again. Like my brother, I couldn't get used to this place.

My prayers were answered four months later when a hand-grenade went off in the empty lot behind our apartment building and my mother declared enough was enough. We were moving to Niger.

Our one-year stint didn't quite work out the way we had originally planned. The initial plan was that we would be homeschooled until we could go back to Pakistan and rejoin our regular schools. Homeschooling turned out to be fun. School but without the yelling students and the finger-pointing and the presentations and the talking? Perfect!

But as the months dragged on and my parents decided to stay on for another year, it was time to put us back in school. Much to my dismay, I ended up right back where I started. More name-calling. More finger-pointing. Add a basketball to the head. Great times. By the time I changed schools again for high school, I had stopped talking. I did make some friends eventually and managed to both settle in and open up, but I never felt a part of the community. I always felt like an outsider, someone who didn't belong there. It had nothing to do with the fact that it was a missionary school and I was, well, not Christian. I simply didn't feel at ease in my skin and around people. Especially so close-knit a community.

By the time graduation rolled around, I had been accepted at the American University of Sharjah in the United Arab Emirates.

A few months after graduation I packed up and in a tearful airport goodbye where in pure Pakistani fashion my entire family came to see me off, I was off to Sharjah to study Interior Design. I think I cried that entire plane ride, and during the transit, and the second plane ride…and the taxi ride to the university campus. And once I arrived at the dorm. I cried a lot basically.

University started off very lonely, and I couldn't reconcile just how expensive it was and how big and how different. Academically I was fine. I was on an eighty percent merit scholarship. I won the Dean's List scholarship every semester. I won both the silver and the bronze Chancellor's Award and was well on my way gunning for the gold. I was in honor's classes. My non-design professors liked me. But in every other way, I was not so hot.

By the time third year rolled around, I was a wreck. I wasn't eating right. My grades had slipped. I wasn't talking in class again. My design work got progressively worse as did my ability to present my thoughts. I realized I wasn't cut out for the design world and the amount of talking and conversing it entailed. Worse, my withdrawn behavior put me at odds with my studio professor. She was one of those people who liked to be told she was super smart and talented, and I refused to indulge. So my grades took the hit and I lost the gold Chancellor's Award by a margin so thin it would take a magnifying glass to see it.

I lost my shit.

I started engaging in self-destructive behavior. Not drinking and partying. No I did the *halal* rebelling. And I declared 'screw you' to the world and everyone in it. Till I got the email from the university counselor's office. Apparently some professor had reported my behavior as unsettling and I was called in for an evaluation. At the risk of them calling my parents, I showed up and took the stupid test, without saying a word the entire thirty-minute session.

The counselor looked over my scrawled answers and solemnly declared that I might actually have Social Anxiety Disorder. S.A.D.

My world crumbled. Shit. I was crazy?! I can understand being called a little odd, but outright crazy?! No way. Not me. Right?

Wrong.

Once I had the term, no matter how much I denied it, I began to see the signs. I avoided people, I feared them. I feared what they thought of me and that obsession with other people's impressions of me dominated my thoughts and actions. I couldn't participate in most normal activities like other people. I was ashamed of the way I was.

I might actually have this social anxiety thing.

And I didn't know how to deal with it.

Once I graduated with my degree in hand, I decided I needed some time off to think of my next steps. I hated interior design, but what could I do that would mean minimal social interaction? And after an intensive search, I came across Cultural Heritage Management. It was related to history like I had always wanted, and if I played my cards right, I could get a job as a researcher or an archivist and wouldn't have to deal with people. It was perfect.

So I applied to Paris for my Master's degree in Heritage and landed a job in Sharjah as a researcher.

But while things were looking up for my life and future career prospects, my mental health kept plummeting and my life and job suffered for it. I was anxious, I was stressed, I was depressed, and I was suicidal.

It was time to find professional help. But professional help, as it turned out, didn't know what to do with me either. Therapy backfired, the medication worked half the time.

My time with professional help was fraught with misunderstanding and strife and confusion. Needless to say, it did not work out.

What was the problem? Why couldn't anyone understand me? These guys were supposed to be professionals. Yet, they seemed just as perplexed by my behavior as I was. What gives?

I tried turning to literature and research studies to try to figure out what was so wrong with me that it warranted the term 'irreparable.' But literature seemed just as confused as my doctors and friends. Some people called it introversion. Others called it shyness. Still others combined terms and called the condition shy introversion. While these are all valid terms, they didn't quite explain *me*. Nothing seemed to fit. And nothing seemed to explain what it felt like to have the condition much less explain why I acted the way I did. Anything that did exist in publication was a mishmash of research studies where researchers told some poor sods like me to give a speech after having their brains mucked with. What is with Social Anxiety research and speeches anyway?

How to cure me began to seem like a far-away dream.

Despite being one of the fastest growing mental illnesses, I realized Social Anxiety Disorder is among the least understood anxiety disorders. And I guess people like me who suffer from it are partly to blame for that. You see, the condition makes it near impossible to tell other people what we are feeling and what we are thinking for fear of getting judged. So we hide it away. We bury our thoughts deep and hide them from the light of day. If we refuse to share how our mind works, it's little wonder that no one understands how it works, isn't it?

So I have decided to grit my teeth and bare my mind, spirit, and soul for all my fellow S.A.D. sufferers out there. What this rabble of half-crazed musings do, or at least try to do, is explain what it's like to live with Social Anxiety. It tries to exhibit why we might do the things that we do. And then it tries to share some of the things that worked for me.

The second half of the book consists of my musings on how to approach Social Anxiety from a therapist's perspective. Not in a clinical research-based kind of way. I think enough of that exists out there. But I try to present what would have worked for me. From a patient's point of view. A patient's perspective, for patients, by a patient. The ultimate in the blind leading the seeing.

I will be so bold as to assume we all want the same thing: to get better. But I realize there are not a lot of resources out there to help us explain to our therapists what we need them to do. And it's not like we are going to say anything, am I right?

So may my thoughts help you find companionship or explain to your therapists or loved ones what's wrong.

Here's to ending our living, waking nightmare.

Chapter One
Self-Consciousness

Tap-taptap-tap-tap, taptap-tap-taptap

The irregular frantic pattern competed with the steady tick of the overly large clock that graced the wall behind the cluttered desk, its jerking second hand a stern understudy of the woman who had yet to appear from the little back room.

The tapping stopped momentarily, replaced by the shuffling of canvas shoes, the whisk-whisk of denim jeans as I fidgeted on the well-worn visitor's chair. Fingers reached up from the depths of an oversized sleeve to pull the hood further forward, aware but uncaring that the need to cover my face had dragged the garment too far up from the back, causing it to hang off the shoulders funny. It's not like it mattered with the number of layers I was wearing. Their job done, the fingers returned to the cold surface of the table. *Tap-tap tap-tap-tap tap*, they started again, an unwanted side-kick to the persistent twitch in my hands, a Morse code I had yet to decipher.

I chewed on my bottom lip and directed my study to the desk instead, an idle attempt to understand the woman I was going to meet shortly.

The melamine veneer on the cheap office desk was peeling off at the edges, the surface of the ugly mottled gray thankfully hidden under the chaos of papers and files and pens and fat unscented candles that seemed to be there for décor more than to serve an actual use. A pen holder rattled slightly against the computer monitor, complaining about the disturbance I was causing it and I quickly moved my contrite hands into the pockets of the hoodie. The clock ticked onward, seemingly louder than before in the ensuing silence.

The notion to knock on the door behind the desk and summon forth the woman who had me waiting for – a quick glance at the clock – 27 minutes now, whined childishly in my mind yet again. My gaze lingered on the door left ajar. Warm yellow light poured lazily out, a welcome contrast to the daunting white of the reception area. I could see the corner of a bedpost beyond the crack. That must be the dorm supervisor's living quarters. Maybe she was sleeping.

Sniff. The incense told me otherwise. The woman was elderly; I could already smell that much.

Get up, idiot.

My knee started bouncing of its own accord, a whimsical dance up and down and up and down and – I stood up quickly to make it stop. Regret tasted bitter in the back of my mouth as my legs protested shakily to what I was asking them to do: take me to the door.

Something settled in my chest, a familiar snake winding itself around my lungs. I swallowed, trying to appease it, enough to at least loosen its grip.

Incense mingled with Arabic coffee. I could smell it now from this close. I reached up to knock but my hands refused to leave their refuge. Fingernails dug trenches into my palm, a futile protest as I forcibly extracted a hand and reached up to deliver the most pathetic knock this dull gray door had probably ever encountered. The thought of knocking again ran to the forefront of my thoughts like an over-exuberant child in gym class. It immediately got the beat down it deserved and I was firmly back in the chair before its cries had died down. As if I had never left my place.

I turned my diligent study to the tiled floor, white ceramic pretending to be marble. The lateness of the hour bled in through the glass of the exterior door like a blanket of black, slithering silently to the corners of the reception area. There was a potted tree beside the door, its branches a natural canopy to the door, but I couldn't see it through the inky black. Only the harsh fluorescent ceiling lights kept the darkness at bay, a little island around the lone desk, and I fervently wished I didn't feel like such a spectacle. There was no one awake at 4 AM, that much I was sure of, but the feeling of being watched crawled up my spine like a spider.

My back ached and the terrible turn of a headache mutating into something worse drummed an angry beat behind my temples. It was violently interrupted by the wailing squeak of a door – a mocking lesson on how to properly announce oneself – and I heard the woman before I saw her, the *slap-thwap* of flip flops declaring when she had made her way to her chair behind the desk.

"Sorry, dearie! You been waiting long?" The lilting accent of the voice painted a picture of a motherly woman in her late forties, wide hips, and an easy smile. My eyes flicked up briefly to confirm the image as I swiveled in my chair awkwardly to half-face her general direction. She looked like she had woken up from a nap, short curly hair askew, the salt and pepper of it glowing softly in the light. Her flowery pink t-shirt just barely hanging on to one shoulder, happily harmonizing with the darks of her skin tone. A glint of gold declared a nose piercing accentuating her features, small eyes crinkled with too many smiles, thin brows and a wide forehead.

Sudanese, the incense declared. Sweet, said the lips. Waiting, said her eyes.

She asked me a question, that's right. I smiled at her to let her know it was OK and I didn't mind the wait.

I did mind.

Her face didn't change and it occurred to me that she probably couldn't see me because of the hood. I shook my head instead and looked up a little so the light would reveal my face. I smiled tightly again.

Liar.

She had already turned away, still smiling, wide and welcoming. A jiggle of the mouse and the monitor flared to life. Light brown eyes. They suited her. She was a shrewd but kind woman.

But I preferred the desk as her fingers took over my role, drumming an irregular beat into the keyboard.

"You must have had a long flight, dear," the woman crooned. I smiled softly at the papers scattered before her. She asked me for my ID and I slid my passport toward her on the desk. Paranoia sparked to life momentarily as she entered my details into the computer. It was restrained just as quickly as it came.

"Oh you have a pretty name," she praised and commenced what looked like a long winded search for something through the jumbled puzzle of her desk top, chatting amicably about something that I had stopped registering a while back.

The mess on the desk suited her perfectly, I decided.

Clack clackitty-clack clack.

The wheels of the ancient suitcase had worn down to the bare plastic after all these years. I hated how loud they sounded against the tiles, hated the way the sound echoed off the walls, hated how long the hall was.

Everything was white. White ceiling, white walls, white floor. White lights that sprung to life as I passed under them. The doors along the walls bore a tired gray, the room numbers illuminating harshly on shiny silver labels as I walked past. 131, 132, 133...

Figures that my room would be near the end of the dorm hall.

Clackitty-clack clackitty-clack clack.

This place looks more like a psych hospital than a girl's dormitory.

Welcome to your new home.

143.

The room card held tightly in my hand confirmed that I was finally where I was supposed to be. The hallway was too exposed, despite the hour. A sharp beep and a green light and the door unlocked.

A little entrance space was the first thing I saw once I found the light switch. A little concrete box that the entrance door swung into and housed the criminally tiny built-in closets. That's going to be real awkward to change clothes here if someone opens the door.

The suitcase struggled over the threshold like an old man and landed in the room with a last heavy thud. The door clicked shut quickly behind it and I stepped forward to see my new living quarters for the foreseeable future. The layout of the room left one of the beds right in front of the door and I immediately decided that was not going to be mine.

The room itself lay beyond the embarrassment zone, a bare necessity affair with two single beds laid out foot to foot, a small bedside table clinging awkwardly besides the too-fat mattress, and a small study desk. One of the desks was conspicuously missing a chair while the other housed a small armless swivel chair tucked in, backrest crooked and the bright royal blue a stark contrast to the place's endless preference for white walls.

A bedsheet and duvet set lay on each bed, waiting like a loyal butler. The light blue one lounged on the bed I had claimed as mine, and guilt tingled in my mouth like a sour orange as I switched it quickly with the green one on the other bed. My fingers started their manic dance again, the feeling of being a thief caught red-handed a red-hot brand in my mind. A little adjustment and the duvet set looked like it had been on the wrong bed all along. A jerk of the head to confirm that no one had witnessed the crime. But the room was just as empty as before, door still closed, the phantom feeling of eyes still present.

Speed became the saving grace, as though the faster the bed spread was set on the mattress, the more it cemented that it was mine to begin with. It was an unfounded concern, the bedspreads were not assigned by name, nor would anyone accuse of robbery over a mere preference of color. Maybe the haste was the need to hide the mattress. I didn't like looking at the surfaces of mattresses. Old habit.

Unpacking the busted suitcase was just as fast, unlike the decision for which wardrobe to claim as mine. The one half behind the door was preferable; the threat of getting smacked by the door miles better than getting caught half naked by whoever happened to be passing in the hallway when my future roommate opens the door.

The thought gave me pause, a screeching halt in cognitive capacity. The empty bed seemed to stare, hostile and promising captivity once its occupant arrived. Not for the first time I wished I had fought harder for the privileged decency of privacy. But finances are a harsh opponent to fight, added to a misplaced parental lament that wailed at the threat of depriving their only daughter of social vibrancy, and it was a conversation that ended before it even started.

I wonder, how long will you last?

The suitcase was laid out on the floor with the gentlest handling it had probably received in years. The fabric around the corners was reduced to threads, fluffy unraveled canvas an absurdly loyal companion that simply refused to give in regardless of how many years of thankless service it had seen. In all honesty, the bag was probably older than I was, a little piece of my personal heritage that had followed me here from halfway across the world.

The neatly placed contents had not moved an inch, a testament to the practiced skill with which they were packed and now transferred to the wardrobe. 10 minutes was all that was needed to unpack my life with a swirling mix of pride and incredulity.

My phone cried out for sustenance, the dulled screen displaying a grim reminder that it was nearly 5 AM and all that remained to do now was wait for the person I will be sharing air with for the next few years. I plugged the practically antique phone into the socket above the side table. It half hovered on its too-short cord like a chunky black TV remote with an oddly orange screen. This phone model had probably stopped being manufactured by the time I bought it, but it was the best option available to me where I lived. The two of us had grown into codependent companions of sorts and as the tired machine settled on its electrical meal, I likewise settled down uneasily on the mattress to wait for nothing in particular.

Lumpy. The mattress had seen too much use, coils digging into bone where it was sunken in.

If you lie down just right, it could be either a massage or a torture rack. Which will you choose?

I shook my head. There were cobwebs growing inside my skull that needed to be shaken loose. I'd slept on worse.

I should probably eat. My last meal was a haphazard picking of bits of stale bun and airplane food. Appetite denied the need, and I dismissed the effort of trying to find something at this hour anyway.

Instead, changing to pajamas seemed a much more appealing idea. Cotton fabric was too light compared to the jeans. The absurd feeling of overexposure in my long-sleeved t-shirt lingered like garlic aftertaste, hastily remedied by pulling the large black hoodie back on over the pajamas and allowing my frame to drown in it.

The phone should last till morning. Lights off.

The duvet was at least warm if not overly soft. Good. The squishy rubber of my earphones found themselves subject to an unwanted massage as I contemplated indulging in some music before bed. The thought ran in circles, round and round and round and round till the only relief was found in firmly plugging the jack in the port on the phone, the click of fingernails on the touchscreen soft as they pulled up the music player. I flicked over to the playlists and scrolled down the obsessively, meticulously, organized list till I landed on the song I was looking for.

Lullabies softly filtered through the ear pieces, little wisps of pearly blue and moonlight silver as my fingers unconsciously wove the melody in the air.

I finally wove my way to sleep, and the rest of the dorm's occupants followed me that night.

Chapter Two
Memory

Memory is a funny thing, isn't it? The ability to bring to your awareness something that happened, or someone you knew, from the past during your waking present. It's a hauntingly beautiful idea. If you can recall something in the present, does that mean the event is still happening, just confined to the dimensions of your mind? If that were true, can an event ever really stop happening?

Is remembrance truly immortality?

Memories can be altered, changed and warped and tainted by just about anything and everything. So if I alter a memory, have I created an alternate universe that only I can occupy?

I digress.

We are told over and over that memory is unreliable, yet we rely on it every day. From remembering the mundane details of how to button up a shirt to remembering a friend's birthday, to remembering a stranger we saw on the bus on the way to work.

Memory guides us. Reassures us.

And in my case, drives us. Mad.

I spend a lot of time thinking about memory. And for very good reason; not to toot my own horn or nothing, but I have a pretty good memory.

I'm not a hyperthymesiac (what are they called anyway?) or anything. But by average standards, your girl here can go toe-to-toe with the best of them.

I can remember textbooks of information after reading them just once. I can remember what someone said to me at a particular moment years after the event has happened. I can remember what someone looked like on a particular day.

I remember events that shouldn't be possible.

I remember the plan of our house when I was barely a year old. I can remember my birthday. My first birthday. I remember my mother doing laundry in the courtyard when I was a wee crawling tyke. I remember a random Sunday as my mother cooked half-fried eggs while my father pushed me on a little red swing that they had hung in the doorway of our dining room when I was still a baby. I remember what my crib looked like, felt like, though thank goodness not smelled like. I remember I had a yellow pair of overalls as a baby, a gentle yellow like the sun at seven in the morning.

I remember, I remember, I remember.

I can remember a dirty look, a gentle word, a kind deed. I can remember something when nothing actually happened. And I can make something to fill that nothing.

Have I lost you yet?

Let me break it down another way.

I remember things about people years after that person is no longer even around me. Such as a conversation I had with a classmate in middle school, or what someone dressed like that one day in high school, or an embarrassing incident someone had on the side of the road that I happened to see from the window of my car. You know, where you see a kid wipe out on a bike and you giggle to yourself and in a moment of utter apathy you mutter, "what an idiot." I remember those moments. And I recall them on occasion, whether on a casual whim or triggered by something around me. Oh, I remember the day when So-and-so came to class dressed in *that* dress. I can't help it. Memories just seem to stick, and they seem to play regardless of whether I want to remember them or not.

But while I may be blessed with a good memory, I am also a firm believer in the knowledge that I am not something out of the ordinary. Like I said, I do not have hyperthymesia. I don't even have a photographic memory. I can't remember something as simple as my cousins' birthdays. Half the time I forget my own. I forget to do the dishes, or feed the cat, or send an email. No, I was born a rather ordinary chubby healthy baby, to a rather ordinary Pakistani couple. By ordinary I mean forced to subjugate to our culture's insistent persistence that anyone who walks this tainted Earth must get married and make lots of babies. Yeah, topic for another chapter methinks.

So stay with me here. If I am ordinary, yet I remember minute details about people on a whim, is it so far out of the realm of possibility or probability that other people remember me and think of me too?

And therein lies the problem.

The possibility of that terrifies me. Rather the inevitability of that crushes me. I am terrified of being remembered more than I am scared of not being remembered at all.

If people remember me, and remembrance is immortality, the idea of leaving the kind of memories others form of me up to chance is unbearable. The very notion haunts my living existence. Because the root of the matter is, I cannot bear the thought of being remembered as weak. Especially considering my condition made me an awkward child and an even more awkward teen.

I said awkward things 'cause uncomfortable silences were too, well, uncomfortable. I had massive breakouts of acne when I hit puberty. I was clingy and whiny, or at least I'm sure I was. I sought attention because loneliness was a torment, but then found that when I had the attention I sought it turned out to be more of a punishment than invisibility. I thought I was creative and had a career as an artistic soul. I had a tummy that stuck out and refused to go away. Needless to say, I am not short of embarrassing and some downright humiliating stories from growing up. At least they are mortifying to me and I would honestly rather die than have someone recount one of those moments. No exaggeration intended. It's been a hard truth to admit that I cannot face the fallible human being that is myself.

Trying to maintain an inerrantly good impression that lasts a lifetime becomes a tricky line to traverse. No. It is impossible, isn't it?

Having achieved some modicum of self-enlightenment in my glorious and wise mid-twenties, I have arrived at a fascinatingly obvious realization: I have no control over how someone from the past remembers me.

Only problem is I am incapable of accepting this as fact and coming to terms with it. That would be the perfectionist in me talking.

I've been told all my life that I am so harsh with myself because I am a perfectionist. That is true, there's no denying that, but I would say that perfectionism is not part of my personality from the get-go. Perfectionism in my case is an aftertaste of social anxiety.

A little bit of perfectionism never hurt anybody. In fact it could really do a lot of good, push your strengths and expand the limits of your capability. But with social anxiety, there are no halfway points with perfectionism. Either every social scenario is utter perfection or I'm a babbling idiot. There's no pass, there is only 100% or a big fat zero.

With that in mind, I cannot leave memory up to chance. No, I must *control* how you will remember me.

This persistent *need* to sculpt the perfect image that is free from the blemishes of judgement and embarrassment has led me down a very solitary path indeed. Cold hard logic, or lack thereof, was my downfall. If you knew me at my perceived worst and I cannot control or alter the image you have of me, then I must never see you again if I am to avoid reliving the shame of how you must remember me: Weak. And stupid.

If I cannot control the memory of me that you already have, I will cut ties with you as soon as the opportunity presents itself. In order to protect myself from repeating the torment that I believe you know.

I no longer have contact with most of my old friends and acquaintances, not because we simply fell out of touch but because I am terrified of the opinion they hold of me. I don't have very many friends as you can see.

Usually when people think of Social Anxiety Disorder, the image that comes to mind is of an awkward misfit character who avoids strangers like the plague. Maybe that is because of the ambiguity between the terms introversion, shyness, and social anxiety. With the way the terms are thrown around, it has become muddier, not clearer, where one range on the spectrum ends and another begins.

Am I a clear-cut textbook example of how a socially anxious person acts? Ha, ha, no. Please. I am a shy introverted socially anxious motherfucker.

In all mock-seriousness, this is probably where my sense of 'wrongness' draws power from. I am as close to fine as is possible for me when I'm around strangers. But I am a wreck with acquaintances.

In fact, interacting with a stranger is far more preferable, since I know I will never meet them again. Strangers on the metro, or on the bus, or on the sidewalk are easier because they are not a risk of validating my fear of being remembered negatively. People that I know I will meet again are a different story. Acquaintances are risky. They are in the process of forming a memory file of how they perceive 'me' and the pressure is on to be absolutely perfect. But even more dangerously so, I will meet them again. They have the opportunity to prove that the fears I hold so tightly in my heart could be real. The fear that I really am a loser, or fat, or ugly, or stupid.

So I go to great lengths to ensure that you will remember me the way I am comfortable being remembered. When it comes to self-introductions, I embellish. With just enough fiction to be believable. With just enough bravado to be enthralling.

So let's play a little game. Catch the fibs that my introduction would contain.

I am a researcher. I studied Interior Design for my bachelor's degree until I realized I didn't enjoy it. I was a good student. I love reading. I once saw a gunman in the stairwell of our Pakistani apartment as he pointed a gun at me. People picked on me as a kid. A hand grenade exploded in the empty lot behind our apartment building in Karachi. I was chubby as a kid and I hate seeing pictures of myself. I once thought my mother was dead in a gas station explosion and I had resigned myself to taking care of my younger brother as an orphan. I love watching TV. I thought I lost my dad and brother in a bomb blast once. I have aspired to be a writer since I was a little girl.

Oh yes, you guessed it. All of those are true. I tell stories of horror and death that I have seen with a smile and casual camaraderie. As if it unfazes me. As if I couldn't be so weak as to have nightmares or anything like that.

Because the truth is, it really doesn't faze me. The lies I face in my own head are more terrifying than whatever life has thrown at me. Yes I had a gunman point a gun at me, yes it scared me. Does it scare me still? No.

But you don't have to know that now do you? Aha, let the mindfuckery begin.

Chances are, if I was introducing myself to you, I would tell you of my sorry tale of woe with the bombs and guns and violence. I would admit that I spend a lot of time being scared. Maybe at some point in my life I was. But what matters now is the performance. The gentle tremble of lips, the hushed voice, the darting eyes.

At this point you must be wondering, and rightly so, what does all this accomplish? That, dear friend, is what I am getting at. This 'performance' as I call it creates the memory of me that I want you to have. I try to create this persona of wonder. I try to make you ponder: how can someone who has been through so much be so strong?

It all boils down to one thing: I am manipulative and I am a liar. Because the memory of the muffintop is what keeps me awake at night, not the guman or the grenade. And that alone is messed up.

Because ultimately, that's the *real* root of the matter. Yes I have suffered, just not in the way I am telling you. But I don't feel strong. I feel weak. And what I am doing is sending a desperate cry for someone, anyone, everyone, to acknowledge the struggle I fight in my head every waking minute of every day. Because maybe, maybe if enough people say that I am truly strong, I will learn to believe it.

So in the hopes of hearing those words, I will mold your memory of me as something so magnificent that not only will you have to remember it, but it will trump the way you remember my muffintop, or my bangs phase, or anything else that I can't stand to face. If memories are immortalizing then at least the version of me that lives on is something good. Because the 'me' I am is the one I want you to acknowledge but never know.

So I must ask you, how will you remember me?

Chapter Three
Judgment

The first time I tried going to a clinical psychologist, he asked me to tell him what was wrong with me. Understandably, this did not go over quite so well in my head. Wasn't it *his* job to tell me what was wrong with me?

I knew what he was trying to do. He wanted to hear me say it, hear my perspective as it were. Inevitably, all my racing thoughts went frantic in a rather familiar but equally unpredictable pattern. *He's going to judge my answer and, being a professional, he's going to think I'm stupid for saying what I'm about to say.* I feel my left leg start to bounce, a habit when I'm nervous. *I'm going to say the wrong thing and he is going to tell me just how wrong I am.* I swallow with great difficulty. It's like my throat and tongue are made from sandpaper. *In his head he's going to laugh at me. Even if he doesn't laugh out loud. When I leave the room he is going to think of the stupid girl who wasted his time.*

Nope, it was decided: I was not going to open my mouth. Which meant bring in evasive tactic number one: Deflect.

"I was rather hoping you would tell me."

Yes, nice save. I mentally high-fived myself while giving myself a hard kick in my mental ass for being such a wuss.

"I need you to tell me first and then I will tell you what I think," he replied.

Isn't that just dandy? He wants to see my living waking nightmare manifested before my very eyes. His answer was exactly what I feared was going to happen, and it did nothing to absolve my rising panic at such a simple request.

I realize you and I probably have very different definitions of simple. The request might be simple in theory, but in practice it was the weighted expectation of it that's hard. I could tell him why I was there, sure. What I couldn't do was hear him 'tell me what he thinks.'

I decided that the evasive techniques were not going to do me any favors. After all, I had become desperate enough to seek professional help. Not getting to the reason why I was there was pointless. The added lightness of my wallet after paying the consultation fees was also a good motivation to open my mouth and blurt out "I think I have social anxiety" in a voice so low it was a miracle he heard it. That shit was expensive, so let the therapy-ing begin.

But that shit I just mumbled was another evasive technique. I didn't think I had social anxiety. I knew without a shred of doubt. I had done my googling (plus I had been diagnosed in college). The technique was evasive because 'I think' took some of the pressure off. It seemed better than outright declaring I had social anxiety. Somehow it felt like if he disagreed he would judge me less with 'I think' as opposed to 'I have.'

My assumption was wrong. The nightmare was just beginning.

"No, I want *you* to tell me," he replied. "Without definitions and terminologies. I want you to explain to me why you are here to see me today."

Well, shit. Was he asking me to define the nature of Social Anxiety Disorder for him? Ha, ha. Easy. Where do I begin?

But I didn't tell him that right away. I didn't want him to think I was some half-assed, half-cocked, guns blazing kind of fool. More importantly, I didn't want him to think I had memorized my answer off of Google or something. And I didn't want him to know that I had rehearsed every possible way this scenario could have gone and that as an introspective old soul, I was wildly aware of the terrible secret that I was going to tell him.

So instead, I take a few moments to look pensive and pretend to think about my reply. I gave it about twenty seconds before I looked in his general direction and answered. The truth this time.

"I let my fear of what other people think of me control me and it's keeping me from living the life I should be living."

The psychologist nodded sagely, approving of my answer. I knew he was going to do that. What I did not anticipate was my own reaction to what I just said.

My eyes welled with tears. There was a tightness in my chest. And before I knew it, I was crying silently, mourning the life that died before I could be living it, and feeling the weight of my statement drain the joy out of my spirit of living.

Because that was ultimately why I had caved and gone to the therapist; I no longer felt the will to live. Why should I? My life didn't feel like my own. Every decision, every action was undertaken depending on how it would make others think of me, even when I know they don't spare me a second thought. I felt lost under the mountain pile of restrictions I had planted on myself for fear of how others perceive me.

The pain of my existence crashed down on me, the pain of every day of struggle and strife and the utter exhaustion of it all.

Because that's what Social Anxiety does: it stops you from living until you're just a husk of a shell, alive but empty.

When I was younger, I often heard the phrase "she's just shy, she will grow out of it." So I waited, but I never seemed to 'grow out of it.' I was still awkward, hiding behind my mother till I towered past her, speaking so low that people stopped trying to interact with me at all because I was so hard to hear. I couldn't make friends, make connections, hold conversations, maintain eye contact. I seemed to embody the irrational and destructive socially-prized Pakistani moral standard of "what will people say?"

And I hated it.

As a child, I couldn't make and keep friends. As a teenager, I felt like I couldn't fit in. As a young adult my stellar academic performance in college slipped (please, of course I had stellar grades, I'm South Asian). And as a working professional, my job suffered. It still does.

Part of the problem, perhaps, lay in the way we use the term shy. Shyness is a personality trait, and declaring that I would grow out of it as if it was some horrible affliction or at best a mildly annoying habit, simply reinforced the notion that there was something inherently wrong with me.

Schools and my parents tried to first convince me that I was simply an introvert. But I guess I must have introverted wrong because eventually the people around me were forced to admit that perhaps I was actually shy. I could feel my parents' disappointment in me, the perceived sense of failure as if I had somehow let them down.

And that there is the key difference between being shy and being socially anxious: the sense of self-instigated failure for being the way you are.

If you'll excuse me, I'm going to turn into a dictionary now for a second. Because the difference between the terms introversion, shyness, and social anxiety need to be hashed out. With the way popular media glorifies the introvert in every wrong way and throws the term social anxiety around, it's little wonder everything has become so muddled.

Am I a qualified professional? No. Am I the best person to be giving out these definitions? Probably not. But hey, these definitions are about my life and having suffered the effects of the meanings, I believe that gives me the right to tackle them. Instead of scientific definitions from the manual of mental health disorders, I'm going to say it as I've seen it. After all, like I said: I'm a shy introverted socially anxious mofo. To paraphrase.

You see, according to the broadly accepted definition, an introvert is someone who draws energy from solitude and introspection. They are like phones. They charge when you leave them alone, and the battery drains when you use them and interact with them. That doesn't mean they don't like being interacted with; they just need their charging time afterward. Don't laugh at me, I'm rather proud of that analogy.

Shyness, on the other hand, is apprehension or aversion to interacting with others for fear of being evaluated by them.

Seems different from introversion? It should be. Shyness is a personality trait. What that means is you're most likely born with it. Psychologists like Dr. Ellen Hendriksen use the term behavioral inhibition.

But here is where things get tricky. Fear of interaction with others, aversion to social situations, and fear of being evaluated by others? Sound familiar? It sounds like there is much overlap between shyness and Social Anxiety. But where do they differ? When does a person stop being shy and become socially anxious?

Here are the differences I have observed in myself that I have not found in people with shyness:

- The level of fear is extreme enough that it becomes distressing or disruptive
- There is a great deal of anguish and suffering whether the feared social situation is attended *or* avoided
- The fear of humiliation negatively impacts daily living and living functions
- There is marked distress about having the condition of Social Anxiety itself

A person with shyness can accept their trait and learn to be content with it. But a person with Social Anxiety will never look at their condition in a positive light. You could say that it is part of what makes the disorder diagnosable. As far as I am concerned, there is simply too much pain involved with having it to be able to accept it, much less be content with it.

It is a flaw in us, it will always be the biggest flaw in us.

Fundamentally, Social Anxiety Disorder is being unable to see ourselves for who we are and believing that the distorted and contorted vision of ourselves we see is the truth. Or perhaps more accurately, it is the fear that others will see it too and reject us for it. Social Anxiety is often labeled as the fear of judgment. I would argue that it is the fear that the judgment we receive is the truth. Dr. Hendriksen calls this the fear of the Reveal, the moment when everyone sees our biggest flaw and collectively shun us for having it.

The other factor that sets Social Anxiety and shyness apart is the level of impact it has on your life.

There is certainly some overlap, but here's the general gist. Shyness can be distressing. Social anxiety will be disruptive.

Allow me to explain using my grades. Because I need some way to make my parents see the value in an A-.

I have always been a model student. Not so much because I studied well and was a diligent little child who cared about her future, but because I was terrified of the humiliation if I did not study hard and was not diligent. I was terrified my parents would think I was dumb.

So, top of the class all around. Every year. Until I got to adolescence and moved to high school.

People were older, they were bigger in general. It was a new crowd and I felt even more like a misfit. It didn't help that it was a Christian missionary school and I was very much *not* Christian. I stopped talking in class, at home. Just stopped talking. Because the terror of being labeled an outcast would be unavoidable if I opened my mouth, because the fact that I was a Muslim, a black fish in a goldfish bowl, would come tumbling out of me if I just talked.

My grades slipped.

It finally came time to pick a career and pick a college and determine my path for the rest of my life. I desperately wanted to pick something in history. But I was told there was no scope or future in that field (heh, future. In history. Get it? Heh) and that was that. I was too scared of rejection and disappointment to fight for it. My grandmother suggested on a whim that I would be good at interior decorating. I figured, why not? I was too scared to actively voice what I wanted anyway and since the idea caught on, I was too self-conscious to say anything against it.

College came. And college kicked my ass. Presentations and reviews and desk-critiques and more presentations and professors with large inflated egos. My grades dropped. I lost my scholarships. I lost my Chancellor's List award. And I lost my remaining self-esteem.

College was probably one of my lowest points. Not only was I struggling miserably academically, but this was the first time I had to live away from home. With strangers no less. It was a perfect recipe for a nightmare.

Although I was lucky enough to bunk with one of my best friends from my second year, the first year was torture. I lived with a stranger, breathed the same air as a stranger, slept in the same room as a stranger. More often than not I ended up doing my homework in the hallways outside the room, feeling miserable and conspicuous as hell against the bare white-ness of the walls and the cold tiled floor.

Food was another nightmare. I was too scared to order in the cafeteria because my indecision over what to get would hold up the line and then where would I be? I was terrified of picking up the phone to call a restaurant and order because first of all, ew phones, and second I was scared they would judge what I ordered. I was too chicken to go to the grocery store and buy food because I feel like the check-out clerk secretly judges the random assortment of things I just bought.

I was too scared to do laundry because what if someone saw me. I was too scared to let the maintenance clean my room because I was scared they would judge the state of my neatness.

At home, your parents deal with everything and you can mooch off the sweat of their brows in happy convenience. On my own, life was stifling and I was suffocating on the vapor of my own fears. Living became a game of daily survival and survival was a game of avoidance.

I took to sleeping in the hallway outside my room because what if I tossed and turned and woke up my light sleeper roommate? I took to memorizing my roommate's schedule and then inhaling any noodles I managed to cook up when she wasn't in the room. I took to going days without food and just dealing with the headaches and hypoglycemia and stomach cramps.

I was slowly killing myself and it took a toll on my body and my mind. I developed a raging ulcer problem and regularly puked up blood in secret and silence. And of course

I was too self-conscious to go to the clinic because what would the doctor think; who gets ulcers at this age?

Most devastatingly, the depression that I had been keeping at bay since I was very young became an unstoppable force and took over every aspect of my life like a tsunami, drowning me with melancholia so severe that there were days breathing was a chore.

Social Anxiety Disorder is the third most common category of mental disorders – at least in the United States – after depression and alcoholism. That's a lot of people for something only a small percentage of the population is said to have. The numbers beg the interesting question of why it is so prevalent.

For one thing, genetics do play a part. Not only is a child more susceptible to developing an anxiety disorder if their parent suffers from it, but it can even be traced back to the beginnings of human ancestry. Back in the dawn of human history, the creation and continued stability of the social unit ensured survival of the group. Any deviance or deviant behavior was punished through isolation. If you threatened the safety of the group, the group isolated the miscreant. Threatening the safety of the group entailed breaking the norms. Losing the approval of the group would certainly mean death. Could Social Anxiety be a remnant from our human ancestors, the hunter-gatherers? Could it be the formed fear of losing the approval of the group that has genetically been passed down through the millenia? Man is, after all, a social animal. So perhaps my theory could have some merit. Someone should really research more into it.

(Not it…plus it's kinda been done, hasn't it? Idiot)

The other part of the puzzle is that Social Anxiety can be a learned behavior while shyness is not; shyness is a personality trait that you are born with. While there is certainly merit in the idea that a past trauma can lead to a person developing social anxiety, I am not ready to believe that it is entirely learned.

Or in a more selfish outlook, there was no event in my life that scarred me so badly that I'm a living breathing wreck of a human being today. By the time the bullies and everything else came around, I had already mastered the art of the socially anxious persona. Where's my trauma that I can blame for all my current troubles?

Truth is, I don't have one. I simply remember being three and thinking to myself that I needed to sit still because what would Mommy think otherwise.

Did I start off as shy and over time develop into Social Anxiety? Perhaps. It would certainly explain the gradual progression of worsening anxiety over the years. Or was I born with all the right genetic code in place to make me grow up loony? I don't know. Hence my socially anxious ape man theory. Someone give me a Nobel Prize please.

Regardless of the root, the effect remains the same I suppose. Judgment and the fear of said damning judgment ran, and still run, every aspect of my day and of my being.

After much evasion, I have to face the truth. I am a coward.

I seem to be stuck in a lake, and for some reason I keep sinking deeper and deeper the more I struggle to break the surface. This analogy too is on point. As I probably should have explained earlier, I can't swim.

To me, it doesn't matter how I ended up in the lake, but what matters is the fact that I am drowning in it. I could weep and whine that there are no hands reaching for me, but the truth is I haven't called for help. Because that would be drawing attention to myself and exposing myself to the risk of people judging me for being in the lake in the first place.

Yeah, I'd rather drown.

Gosh, what you must think of me.

Perhaps I'm just a classic text-book people-pleaser.

For all social anxiety's symptoms, I have never come across people-pleasing as a valid symptom, so maybe it's just me. See, I think there's merit to my theory that most socially anxious people are people-pleasers as well.

Social Anxiety is the fear of negative judgment. Using the theory of elimination, can this mean that socially anxious people would want positive judgment? Is it approval they seek, or do they really want to just be left alone?

A lot of people-pleasing symptoms could match what socially anxious people feel or do. They avoid conflict because it's confrontational and they don't like that. Or pretending to like things others like or agreeing with them because you don't want them to think you are stupid for thinking otherwise. You can't say no because you're scared others might think you are stupid for believing in what you do. Or perhaps you are scared others might think you're selfish for refusing to do a task that's asked of you. You refuse to admit when your feelings are hurt because you're scared someone might think you're weak or being unreasonable. Perhaps you apologize often. I know I am guilty of this one a lot. Seriously, the Canadians would be proud of me. Invite me to your country please.

Or perhaps you feel the burden of what other people want or expect from you and you're scared of disappointing them because then they would leave you.

I know I am guilty of that one too. My hijab is a good example of that. When I decided to wear the scarf, I thought it was what was expected of me. I thought I would make my parents proud by suggesting it before they told me to do it anyway when I was older. As I grew up, I regretted the decision. The approval didn't last long and I came to realize that I had put it on too young. I didn't get to enjoy the freedom I had until I had given it up, subservient to an expectation that I only *thought* was expected of me.

When I later told my parents that I put on the scarf because I thought it was what they wanted, they denied it. Said it was my own decision.

Gosh how quickly approval fades.

Chapter Four
Self-Deprecation

I remember a day when I was in high school, casually sharing a seat with a classmate under a shady tree on some wicker chairs enjoying the afternoon breeze and discussing who in our class would be which Disney princess. You know, regular mature and meaningful conversation. Julie would be Belle of course. Eli would be Snow White because she loved to sing. Ashley would be Aurora. And in all seriousness, I casually declared that we had our Beast. My partner in this pointless act leaned forward, bemused, expecting me to name a boy in our class or something. She was rather shocked when I patiently told her that I was the Beast of course. A moment of silence followed. Which then dragged on. And then on some more. Until my friend finally asked what was on her mind.

"Why do you do that? Why do you always put yourself down?"

Now I could have realized that I had messed up. That my insecurities were showing and it was making people uncomfortable. Future me would have laughed off the tension with some half witty quip about how 'Beast was the best character and how a girl literally fell into his lap while he didn't have to lift a finger, am I right.' But past me was young and naive and so she told the truth as it was.

"Because that's what I am. A Beast."

The mood plunged like a rock in an icy lake.

I was never invited to lunch again.

Do you know Will Poulter? The actor from the Maze Runner movie? Or that other basically porno movie about the Millers or something?

Or better yet, Ryan Reynolds. Yeah I should have led with him.

Stupid.

Do you know what they both have in common?

Their sense of humor. I don't mean they both crack the same jokes, but they both have a self-deprecating style of humor. They put themselves as the butt of the joke while lifting others around them up. It's quite a chivalrous skill. And a difficult one to balance. Because it's one thing to willingly allow others a laugh at your expense (I have no idea how they do it without bursting into tears) and it's quite another to make everyone around you uncomfortable. And with self-deprecation, it's very easy to do the latter.

You can tell where I'm going with this can't you?

Yep! I fall in the latter category! Yay!

OK fine, that's not strictly true anymore. But neither am I in the glorious company of Masters Poulter and Reynolds. Ha! I wish.

A standard Oxford definition of self-deprecation means to be modest about or critical of oneself, especially humorously so.

Not to be immodest or anything but modesty comes easily to me. I'm really rather good at it. Heh, heh.

It's not necessarily a personality trait I was born with, although I suspect it has more to do with the fact that I can't figure out how to react to praise or attention so I avoid highlighting an accomplishment where possible. Is that modesty? Eh, close enough.

Critical about oneself? That I can do. With relish and gusto.

The part about it being humorous? Now that is difficult to pin down. My humor certainly is self-deprecating, but there's a catch. I'm not trying to put myself down to lift someone else up; I'm simply putting myself in my place.

For me, it's not a question of humility. It's about value. And I truly, genuinely believe in the absolute worthlessness of my value to society, to my job, to the people around me. I am not a good friend, or a good daughter, or a good sister, or a good employee. I'm too preoccupied in my own head to be of any external value.

I feel like I am constantly in need of rescue. I am always a ringing phone away from having a meltdown, or a business meeting away from making a fool of myself.

When I moved to Sharjah, I was lucky enough to find a place close enough to one of my best friends. Even more lucky, exactly halfway between both our houses was a Tim Hortons. It was a solemn pact between us that if any one of us had a bad day, we just had to say the word and we would descend upon the poor Tim Hortons like vultures and spend a couple hours just talking and hashing things out. 99% of the time, it was me calling for a Tim's Session, as we called it, because someone asked me a question in a meeting and I screwed up the reply. More often than not, I felt guilty for constantly asking for help when I did not deserve it. And I felt worse about dragging my friend out and wasting her time. Granted there was delicious coffee involved and now we are both addicts of the iced cappuccino.

With my other best friend (not the one I was roommates with in college or the one with the Tim's Sessions – this one's the last one, I promise) we actually came up with a code word to help me get past my feelings of worthlessness and ask for help. Because I would be too self-conscious to ask for help when I needed it, the codeword was something I could just throw out there without overthinking things like I usually do. Our codeword was KOKA. Like the cup noodles. The codeword didn't help, I still ruminated over the prospect of reaching out and wasting somebody's time. But again, more often than not it was me using the bat signal. Everyone else just seemed to have their lives together.

See what I mean when I say I'm in constant need of rescue?

When my friends didn't work out all the time, I created an alter ego to chat with. Not like a D.I.D. alter ego, more like an imaginary friend if I'm perfectly honest. I never had one as a child, figured I'd see what the craze was about.

Her name is Ravenniel and she is everything I could never be. For most of the time, she became someone I could talk to. But only on occasion, as I tend to look like an idiot muttering to herself when I'm talking with Ravenniel, and goodness gracious me if anyone was to ever catch me acting like a lunatic.

Which is probably exactly what I sound like right now. A crazy person talking to made-up alter egos. Believe me, I'm aware of how crazy I sound.

Besides Ravenniel, there's that familiar little voice in my head that constantly yells profanities at me. Reminding me that I am useless and worthless.

I have a tendency to constantly put myself down. Most people have this little voice that comes out in bad times. They can't help it.

That's not me. What makes me ultra-special crazy is that I belittle myself consciously and on purpose. That little voice is me, not some unconscious part of my brain. I employ that voice regardless of whether it is a good situation or a bad one.

You see, my tendency to self-deprecate stems from my sense of failure. I feel like a failure because I cannot overcome something as fundamentally basic as a chemical imbalance in my brain. I am helpless to the force of my fears. So, by what right could I claim the rights of being human if I can't even human right?

When I decided to give therapy a try, I went to several different doctors before I found the one that made me less uncomfortable than the rest. One of the early ones that I visited asked me whether I had thought about marriage or if I had a boyfriend.

"No, I would really like to not get married," I told her.

To my utter confusion, the woman breathed a sigh of relief. "Good," she praised. "Because that wouldn't be fair to the other person now would it? What with you being you."

That stung. Ouch. Harsh.

But not wrong. I mean she could have been less of an ass about it, but ultimately I have to acknowledge that what she said was true.

It is probably one of the base reasons for why I never want to marry. Not only am I terrified of the idea of sharing every intimate detail of my life with another human being, forever, but I don't believe I would be fair for my husband. And that thought alone makes me maddeningly unhappy.

The psychiatrist that I ended up with took a more gentle approach with me. In one of our sessions he asked me what I thought was the point of life. The question stumped me. I gave him a snarky reply about how the point was that there was no point and we are all hurtling towards abysmal oblivion. He smiled slightly at my sarcastic genius and told me that the point is to be happy.

But what if I don't deserve that happiness? I am of the old-fashioned and irrational school of thought that believes that happiness is earned. And I don't feel like I have earned the right to be happy.

It's a delicate line between self-deprecation and self-pity. Quite often I found my self-deprecation leads to self-pity.

Remember the friend I had my doomed lunch with? Yeah I put her through a lot. Shortly after the Beast incident, the two of us signed up to go on a charity mission out to a far-flung rural village to build desks for the local school. We spent a weekend building wooden desks with metal frames and varnishing the desktops and generally having a good time. Yep, even me. Aren't you proud?

When night fell, the rustic little village with its straw huts and animal pens disappeared into pitch blackness. And the whole place was lit by starlight.

I have never seen so many stars in my life! The little village of Inatés was so far away from civilization and had no access to electricity. In short, the sky was clear and oh my word I cannot begin to explain the sheer beauty of the naked night sky. Hues of pinks and purples and clusters of delicate silver lined the silky trail of the Milky Way. I counted nine shooting stars in the span of a couple hours.

A campfire crackled to keep away the November chill. And in the midst of all this wondrous beauty my friend muttered about how she felt people look at her funny.

And I snapped.

For a couple glorious days, I was far from civilization. I didn't feel the constant prickle at the back of my neck as if someone was watching me, or the maddening itch I get when I am around people that makes me want to scratch my skin off. This was as close to freedom as I had ever gotten. And the weight it lifted off of me was beyond belief. I felt lighter, unbound, like a helium balloon released into the sky to go higher and higher and higher. I was drunk on freedom and the sheer release.

And it suddenly sunk in that I had to go back to that damned civilization in the morning. No more freedom. It was back to the feeling of being watched, back to the unbearable strain, back to the constant itch. I suddenly felt like Atlas, pinned under the tremendous weight of my sanity again after having the burden removed for a few tantalizing hours.

I had to go back to my never-ending torment. And what, *she* felt like people looked at her funny? Honey, you don't even know what that means. I do.

And I began to cry. None of the pretty princess crying either. I *cried*. Large guttural sobs that wracked my whole frame and vibrated in my bones. Snot running, tears staining, hiccupping ugly crying and I couldn't stop. I crawled into my tent that I shared with said friend and cried my heart out.

I cried for myself with utter abandon. And for the first time, I truly pitied myself.

Chapter Five
Lies

I followed the therapist into the elevator. My legs were shaking, my clenched fists even more so, the skin of my knuckles stretched white with the strain. My fingernails dug little crescent trenches into my palms, the pain a welcome comfort and a great distraction from what was happening around me.

The therapist strode all the way to the back of the elevator and leaned against the handrail. I wanted to follow her to the back but decided she would not let me pass this test if I did that. So I hovered in the center, leaning against the wall to hold myself up.

The test itself sounded simple enough to anyone else; all I had to do was ride in a crowded elevator to the top floor and back. Easy. Right?

Wrong.

Not for me.

A gaggle of people (that's what they're called right?) sauntered in after us like they owned the place. A man with crutches and a cast on his leg hobbled past me to stand in the back next to the therapist. My breath caught in my throat and I felt the familiar tightening of my chest as if my lungs were being compressed. Oh no, not again, not here!

Too late.

Pain blossomed behind my ribcage and I found I could no longer draw breath as my throat closed up. My legs began to shake harder.

More people piled into the clinic elevator: a pregnant lady, an elderly couple, a young woman, and two tall African dudes (not stereotyping or nothing, their shirts were Senegalese).

The space got cramped and my skin began to prickle on my arms. If I wasn't already shaking so hard I'd be scratching the living daylights out of my skin. I tried to breathe in and follow the breathing technique the therapist was trying to teach me.

The elevator door dinged closed and I flitted my eyes up to realize no one had pressed the top floor button. Of course they hadn't.

I looked over at the therapist for a clue on what to do but she purposely seemed interested in the elderly woman's culottes and refused to make eye contact with me. Did she expect me to ask someone to press the button for me? Or push past the Senegalese man to do it myself? 'Cause LOL, lady neither of those options was happening.

I swallowed.

The elevator started to move.

It was hot. Was it hot? Or was it cold? It was definitely uncomfortable.

The doors dinged open and a middle-aged lady climbed in. She was clad in a bottle-green velvet blazer and she was breathing heavily as if she was in massive pain.

And I choked. Air decided it didn't like the confines of my lungs and went adios amigo. I clutched the handrail for support and focused on trying not to make any noise. This had blown into a full-fledged panic attack and I felt like an absolute moron.

This woman in front of me was in real pain. The guy with his leg in a cast probably was too. What if one of the elderly couple was dying? Not sure what the Senegalese men were doing, they just chatted in French about a cafe they both liked. Maybe they had a sick friend they were visiting?

Point was, these people had real problems in their lives. And here I was making a fuss about a problem that doesn't even exist. No one was even looking at me.

I hiccupped as I tried to breathe through my mouth, an awful gargling choking sound. The Senegalese men stopped talking for a second to glance in my direction. Even the lady in the blazer gave me a look, then tsk'd and looked away again.

See?! I felt halfway validated that people do notice me and think "What an idiot." The therapist's exercise in proving to me nobody paid me a second's notice was wrong! I knew it. I *am* an idiot.

My lungs burned and tears leaked out of my eyes. Oh shit. Not now, not now, please!

I felt humiliated enough already.

I wanted to wipe my tears before anyone noticed them, but at the same time I didn't want to call attention to myself. I felt helpless.

More tears came, not because of the pain in my chest this time. I was honest to God crying now.

So, I just settled for hanging my head as low as I could so no one would see my face. And just focused on riding out the rest of this elevator test. People came and went and I tried to ignore how *loud* everything sounded. The whish-whish of denim fabric, the swish of an abaya, someone scratching their head, a cough, clearing throat. It all pounded against my head.

When the elevator opened onto our floor and the therapist stepped out, I nearly face-planted. My legs were so weak and lifeless. The therapist didn't even look at me, I could tell she was disappointed in me. It took nothing but the sheer force of will to get my legs moving again, encouraged by the thought that if I stayed in there then more people were going to board and I would relive this nightmare all over again.

I was still crying when we entered the therapist's office and we took our seats again, her at her desk, me in the patient's chair.

"Stop crying!" she barked.

I flinched and started crying harder.

In another part of town, a delivery man waited in the elevator as it opened on the eighteenth floor. He looked up from where he was leaning against the wall to curiously peer at who entered. His curiosity was not disappointed. A young woman entered and pressed the button to close the door. She seemed in her mid-twenties but carried herself with poise. She was dressed in an office outfit: cigarette gray pants, a black ruffled shirt, a black hijab and a black and white checkered blazer. Little gold buckles on her shoes and a leather bracelet on her wrist. She seemed as confident as she dressed. What really caught his attention was the box she was carrying by a handle. He moved aside and pulled his two-wheeled delivery dolly to give her some space. She smiled politely but the movement jostled the box and it emitted a weak little mew. She immediately raised the 'box' to her face and shushed the little kitten in the carrier.

"Hush, it's only for a little while," she told the kitten. Her voice was gentle.

"Miaow!" the delivery man cried exuberantly, his attention entirely focused on the carrier now. The young lady laughed and held up the carrier higher so the man could play with the kitten inside. The creature swatted gently at his dancing fingers, the man giggling with glee like a child. "What a nice baby!" he crowed.

"Thank you!" the lady replied. "She's going to the vet for her vaccinations today."

"Ah. In my country we don't have the time to care about cats like that."

"Where are you from?"

"Cameroon."

Her eyes lit up. "I lived in Cameroon for a while! Don't ask me where; I was too young to remember at the time. But I do remember it was beautiful."

The man beamed with joy.

The elevator stopped and opened to let them out on the ground floor. The lady held the door open for the man as he struggled with the dolly.

"It's nice to meet someone who lived in my country," he remarked. "Don't cry when you get your injections, kitty!"

He waved at the kitten once more, then smiled at the lady. And with that the two parted ways.

Would you believe that the person in the two stories is the very same?

No, not the man, the young lady.

It's OK, read them again. I'll wait.

Done?

Now don't misunderstand, this isn't a before and after scenario. I didn't go from a panicking monkey to a dancing one. This isn't an advertisement for how therapy and a go-getter attitude can cure you I'm afraid. I simply learned evasive tactic number three: Lie.

Or as you probably know it better, fake it till you make it.

I was very young when I learned that there is no place in the world for people like me.

I was seven years old and had just moved to the shiny fancy new school in Sudan for third grade. Since this school was further away from our house, I had been handed over to the area school bus to drive me to and from home. One particularly fine summer day, I was running a little late at the end of the day and was the last person to make it to the van. I was embarrassed and mortified at the tardiness. So much so that I settled in for the long ride home on the hard ledge behind the driver and passenger seat, thinking that it was nothing less than I deserved for the delay I had caused everybody. As it happened, everyone else seemed to feel the same way. Nobody offered me the empty folding seat and the bus driver hrumph'd and slid the van door shut forcefully the second I was into the bus. Only problem was, I wasn't all inside the bus. My hand was still holding the frame as I pulled myself into the van. And the door slid into its place with a bang, with my finger sandwiched neatly in the frame. I gasped quietly, the only outward indication that announced the flaming red-hot pain that shot through my hand. I looked mournfully at the bus driver's retreating back, desperately wondering if I should, if I could call him back to open the door for a brief moment and allow my finger to escape. But the shame of my lateness still lingered on my tongue like a sour popsicle, and I found I could not find the courage to call out either in pain or in earnest. And so I sat there for the twenty-minute bus ride, my finger firmly latched in place and dreading every jolt and pothole and jump where the finger would be jiggled from its position. By the time I finally got home, my hand was delicately blue from the restricted blood flow, the digit swollen and blackened with bruises and door grease. As soon as the bus ground to a halt with a last jolt and the door slid open with taunting ease after the pain it put me through, I was out like a rabbit from a burrow during a hunt, my hand clutched tightly to my chest. My eyes misted, both in pain and in shame at my inability to tell someone on the full bus of fellow human beings that "Oh I do say, it seems my finger has been caught in this here door, how silly of me. Could any of you chaps kindly set me free?" *What was wrong with me?* The thought flew in tireless circles in my brain. And not for the first time in my young life did I wonder whether something was truly wrong with me. It was the first time I had to accept the harsh lesson that yes, there was indeed something not quite right upstairs.

My second harsh lesson came soon after the first in the form of a pencil stabbed into my left palm. Remember those pencils where you could pull out the tip once it goes blunt and stick it in the back of the pencil, revealing a brand new sharp point? A few weeks after the finger-in-the-bus incident, I was invited to a birthday party. As all birthday parties tend to do, there was no shortage of games to prove who could memorize the best, or who could run around chairs the fastest, and who could pin tails on a donkey while blindfolded. Being the memory prodigy that I am, I had just won the memorization game where you are shown a box full of random items and the person who remembers the most items in the box wins. A brand new shiny pink pencil was my coveted prize and this fat little chubbabubba of a meatball was rather jealous of it. In a fit of childish rage he stomped over and demanded I give him the pencil. Startled, I looked around for an adult close by who could come to my aid. Naturally there was no one. "No," I choked out finally.

"Give it!" the boy demanded, cheeks puffed and eyes practically bugging out of his head.

I shook mine emphatically no, desperately clutching my prize behind my back, as if that would somehow keep it safe. It was a tactic that didn't work as intended as the boy lunged for me and my pencil. We tussled on the ground for a moment before the boy ran out of breath.

"You're stupid!" he shouted. "You're so fat and stupid!"

Hurt by his words, I held out my prize as a peace offering. I couldn't understand what I had done so wrong to warrant such a tirade of verbal abuse and I hoped that by giving him the pencil he would take back his accusation.

The boy grabbed the pencil and with little warning swung the pencil at my face. On pure reflex, I threw up my hands to protect myself, only to catch the sharp point of the lead in the palm of my hand. The pencil stuck there, and we both looked on in horror as the pink barrel quivered slightly as my hand trembled.

"That's for being stupid," the boy declared in a shrill voice, trying to cover up the fact that he fucked up and he knew it. And off he sauntered, pencil forgotten in my hand, quite literally. No one came to my aid. I just stood there clutching my hand wondering whether I should cry to get someone to come help me. But gosh, I didn't want to be a bother. That evening as I sat on my porch, my mom trying to surgically extract the shards of lead from my hand with a pair of tweezers to the soundtrack of my howling sobs, I pondered what I had done so wrong that not only was I punished by my peers, but was left by the adults to suffer in silence. All I thought I had done was try to pacify the situation and offer a token of peace. Ultimately, I had to face the realization that the world was not made for people like me. It was not built to run on my quiet ideals and timid temperament. I would have to face the lesson that the world was not going to accept me as I am. Try as my mother might, the pencil lead refused to leave the bloody hole in my palm. Till this day I have a small black spot on my left palm, a solemn reminder of my grim lesson.

Thump-thumpthump-Smack!

The little fists pounded against my back and I hunched down further where I sat on the floor. The assembly hall buzzed with excited chatter and the general noise of several hundred students crammed into a single space. The third graders, myself included, sat cross-legged on the floor at the front of the hall. The principal was talking, a long-winded monologue about how he was proud of every grade and every student there for putting forth exceptional effort this year and how it was his joy and honor to present the award for most outstanding student in each grade level. I wasn't listening, my own attention wholly preoccupied by Alison, the girl who was punching my back. Now that I look back on it, I don't really remember where Alison was from. Maybe she was British. Maybe she was American. She was foreign though, clearly demarcated by her bob-cut blonde hair and fair skin and blue eyes. She was the darling of the third grade, a crystal in a handful of pearls. And she was mean. Alison lived in a world of entitlement, the girl destined to be the tippy top of the third grade pyramid. At least until I came along and deposed her from her throne. I was the new teacher's darling, a model student and a well-loved part of the teacher community. So when I won the most outstanding student of the year award in the third grade, Alison took it as a final insult to her pride. She burst into tears and hammered her little fists into my back, a puny childish attempt to regain some of the dignity she was irreparably losing by hitting me. I clutched my prize closer to my chest, a big white hardcover book of *101 Science Experiments to Try at Home*. The girl next to me gave me a rueful sideways glance, clearly sorry for me but unwilling to stick her neck out to help. It was every girl for herself whenever it came to Alison. And so I endured, quietly taking the punishment and wondering where on earth my teacher Mr. Robert had gotten to if he wasn't going to step in and do something.

Assembly finally sang its way to a close with all the students filing out of the main door and heading to our respective classrooms to pick up our stuff and call it a year. I grabbed my backpack, neatly putting my hard-won and much endured prize in my bag next to the lunchbox. A light tap on my shoulder called for my attention, and I turned to see the girl who had been sitting next to me during assembly. She still had that rueful look about her, apology shining in her eyes. "Congratulations," she muttered softly. She couldn't seem to meet my eyes, which was fine by me to be honest. I smiled at her, both accepting her felicitations and letting her know I understood her reluctance to come to my aid in the assembly hall earlier. "Mr. Robert is looking for you. Behind the assembly building." And with that she was off, sprinting away like she was trying out for the sports team. I left my bag and headed outside to the big building where the school met for assemblies. Even as I rounded the corner I never saw the stick coming. It took me by surprise as I felt the hit across the back of my shoulders and lost my balance. The next hit got me behind my knee and sent me sprawling on the ground, only to be reintroduced to the stick across my back. I scrabbled against the dirt trying desperately to find my footing and run away until the stick acquainted itself to the side of my head and sent my vision reeling and my sense of balance out the window. The stick fell, again and again and again and again. Alison was screaming something and a small part in the back of my mind put the pieces together. Of course, it was so simple now! Mr. Robert had never sent for me, but Alison had. And I'd waltzed right into her ambush. *Thwack-thwack-thwack!*

Suddenly, I heard a sharp crack and my first thought was that that was my spine. I tried to wiggle my toes fearfully, terrified that Alison had permanently broken me. My toes moved; so well in fact that I managed to get my legs under me and hobble away around the assembly building and into the playground. I breathed heavily, not aware that I was sobbing, though with pain or with shock I do not know. My uniform dress was ripped and my scattered mind strung itself together to form the coherent thought that my mother was going to ask questions. A few dark stains were spreading through the blue fabric. Blood. I was actually bleeding. There were going to be questions for sure. I didn't even realize I was in the art room until I caught the sharp smell of oil paints and realized I was smearing red paint over my dress in an attempt to cover up the stains. Yes, this could work; I could say I spilled paint in art class. I didn't even realize I was openly crying until my vision blurred and snot blocked my nose. As the bright red paint dried, a harsh lesson worked itself into my mind. The world had no place for quiet butterflies like me.

As I stepped up to the front of the meeting hall, every eye following my most miniscule movement, my persona carefully crafted and well in place, I couldn't help but wonder how I would manage this exercise if I were to do this as my true self. Right now, I was channeling confidence and self-assuredness with all my might and it was draining me as fast as bluetooth drains a smartphone battery. I clasped my hands in front of me, drawing a deep breath to steady my nerves. Before I could allow myself more time to overthink I began as loudly as I could. "The Making of Mankind, By Richard Leaky…"

I gestured the heck out of the presentation, I voice modulated, and I enunciated. Every part of my presentation was perfect and I knew it. Because with long years of practice came the skill of falling into character the way a surgeon's hand slips into a powdered latex glove. And I was playing the audience of twelve at this little High Impact Presentations training course like a fiddle. They stood enthralled by my performance, eyes riveted to my every move, lapping up the words I read out as if the very sounds that came out of my mouth were gospel. The more I spoke, the more ingrained my lesson became; like my boss who sent me to this training course in the first place, every person in the room valued the same thing. They all valued the loud and the bold and the confident. And I relearned a lesson I learned a long time ago: the world valued the loud. And in order to be successful, you *had* to be loud.

"You need to grow out of this now, *beta*."

"The world is going to eat you up."

My parents were well-meaning, I'm sure. But their methods taught me that the world valued the loud and exuberant and in-your-face. It also taught me that there must be something wrong with me if I just couldn't seem to grow out of *it*. Whatever it was. But I have carried the weight of that failure with me all of my life.

When I grew a little older and started school, my *it-ness* made me a magnet for trouble. And I learned my fifth fundamentally important lesson. The world is never going to change. Although Susan Cain tried with her book, *Quiet*, I don't believe the world really changed all that much. All it did was make 'introvert' the new hipster trend. People didn't understand the introvert any better, but they were happy enough to use introversion as an excuse for antisocial behavior. *I don't feel like seeing you today? Oh I must be an introvert.* All that happened was that terms like anxiety no longer became as taboo as they used to be and wound their way into the common vernacular. "Oh my God I hate salesmen; they give me anxiety" became as prevalent as "Oh my God let's eat already; I'm starving." We are lucky enough to not know what starvation is, just like most people are fortunate enough to not know the true horrors of an anxiety disorder. While at its core I am glad mental illness is no longer as taboo as it used to be, having it become mainstream did not help people like me. I won't lie, I judge the heck out of people who "get anxiety" from rather everything. And I cannot bear the thought of stepping out into *this* world, this world of anxiety-ridden people and where depression is treated like the common cold of mental illnesses, and admit that I suffer from anxiety and depression. Knowing that I judge others, I cannot risk the fact of someone else judging me for the same thing. As far as I am concerned, the Quiet Revolution didn't change anything for me. The world went from one extreme to the other and I still do not feel like I can share my rather special struggle with Social Anxiety. The world to me is still as closed off and far away as it ever was. The situation and context may have changed, but the world never did.

In college, I saw the socially adept people succeed regardless of their academic achievements or skill. People who could barely draw a straight line were getting all the professors' attention and all the internship opportunities. The key was networking, something I avoided as if the very mention of the word would cause me to spontaneously combust. But the lesson screamed loud and clear; to succeed in this world, you have to navigate the social sphere. It is unavoidable. Just like standing in the sun is going to get you tanned (yo, I'm desi, we don't sunburn we just darken). It is a lesson I have been forced to relearn at my job. I sat back and watched myself be drawn into and out of office drama as it suited people's whims and wishes. I saw people work their way into positions of ever greater power and influence while I sat in my forgotten little corner and buried my nose into yet another decades old archive. The world is unavoidable and the more you run from it, the more it forgets you exist. The greater your role as a pawn in someone else's game.

I learned my final lesson when I was sent to the counselor's office for an evaluation. The world will never forgive me, and people like me, for being as I am. All we do by acting like we are wired to be, is draw attention to ourselves and invite the judgment of "What a weird freak," that very same judgment we were trying so hard to avoid.

So I can't be me, I can't be successful being me, and to be successful, I have to be not-me? Fine.

This realization awoke two things in me: spite and fear.

Fear, because what if someone found out that I'm on the verge of a meltdown all the time? Any chance of success or a shot at a normal life would be gone. I would be labeled the weirdo and the freak, just like I didn't want to be. What if people found out I was actually a freak? I wasn't helping matters by drawing attention to myself having panic attacks and not talking at dinner parties, or in class, or at work. A condition that is supposed to make me invisible was actually broadcasting itself through behavior that is out of the norm. In order to not mingle with the crowd, I would have to mingle with the crowd.

Spite, however, gave me the strength to do that. I decided I would give the world what it wanted. I would fake it till everyone thought I had made it. I would pretend to be as social or as confident as the situation called for so I can comfortably fly under the radar and not single myself out.

So I carefully crafted a strategy. Or an image or persona as it were.

Luckily as a shut-in I watch a lot of TV. Movies, shows, anime, you name it. And TV is full of characters that people liked. Why couldn't I be one of them?

Well, there was nothing stopping me. So become them I did.

I carefully crafted my personas, each tailored to fit the situation that it will be used in. The confidence of this anime character, mixed with the sense of witty humor of this movie character, with the unassuming sweetness of that one minor character in a book I read once, all mixed with some sugar and spice and everything people liked.

At my parents' desi dinner parties, I was polite, charming, confident, modest, and a jack-of-all-trades. I was Alphonse from Fullmetal Alchemist, Sam from Supernatural, and literally any protagonist from any anime 'cause son they can do anything and everything.

At work I was professional, casually funny, passionate, and calm. For a presentation I was cold and knowledgeable, I was Kaiba from Yugioh (don't diss that show, it was your childhood and you know it).

With delivery-men and sales people, I pretended to be Ravenniel.

With little demons – I MEAN CHILDREN – I was gentle and patient and funny and full of wonder. I was basically Barney.

The point is I stopped being me: shy, unresponsive, anxious, nervous, fidgety, hiding in corners, untalkative, a loner.

And the sad part is, it worked. When I was young, the question I heard the most after "what is your name?" and "how old are you?" was "Do you have a tongue?"

"Can you talk?"

"Is she normal?"

That one was said to my parents.

But the point is I attracted attention I didn't want by the simple act of being me. Once I started putting on my little acts, I stopped getting those questions. No more "Do you even talk at all?"

I'm not saying I'm a complete success. I mess up sometimes.

Goodness knows, when I started it was awkward and painful. My first few 'performances' as I call them were awful. But over time I got the hang of it. It didn't take as long to craft a persona, and it became easier to slip into character. I could keep up the act for longer. Be more convincing.

The technique has helped me land and keep a job, get some friends, have a good rapport with my old professors, order food at restaurants, and so much more. What I am is an actress, and wow did I miss my calling. Should have become an actress in Hollywood. Oscar over here, please!

But the technique is not perfect. It does come with its share of flaws. And I'm talking fundamental flaws.

For one, it is unpredictable. Every situation requires careful planning and strategy. It requires you to understand the kind of people you would be interacting with, knowing what they would like in a person. That works for regular performances like at the office or with acquaintances. But what about situations where you are going for the first time? Or you don't know about anyone there? It's a gamble. Sometimes the persona plays off. Other times I realize I have miscalculated. Knowing what to do then is the real challenge. Do I stick to the planned persona or do I improvise on the spot?

Second, it is taxing. It requires effort, and I mean a lot of effort and energy to keep up the act. The longer the event, the greater the recharging time afterward in the silence of my own company. Told you I was also an introvert.

But perhaps the most prominent of drawbacks is this: I am lying.

And the guilt of that tears at me. Everyone who knows me, knows a lie. The person they know doesn't exist.

And the part that kills me is if they knew the real me, I wouldn't trust them to stay with me. People didn't stay before I started putting on performances. What could lead me to believe that anything would be different this time around?

Look at my pitiful existence. How could you ever leave me?

But then again look at what I'm telling you; how could you possibly stay?

My best friends and family are not people I should be putting on performances for. But I do. Because it makes them leave me alone as well. If I'm chatty at home, everything is fine. If I am my regular quiet, withdrawn self, I keep getting asked what's wrong or why I am sad. I'm not. That's just the real me.

My best friends are worrying. Did I play a character when I got them to be friends with me? Am I still playing one when I'm around them? Is it really me or has the character become so much a part of me that I slip into it without even realizing it? Are they even really friends with *me*? If I acted like the real me now, would they still want to be friends with me? Am I lying to them, manipulating them into being my friends by being a person they would like?

I don't know.

Most people with Social Anxiety engage in one of two behaviors: avoidance or endurance. According to Dr. Hendriksen, avoidance is the kill-switch that turns everyday anxiety and shyness to Social Anxiety. Avoidance is the fuel through which Social Anxiety sustains itself. Avoidance is the long game through which we try to postpone the inevitability of the fear that somehow, someday everyone is going to find out our dirty little secret: that we are flawed, ugly, unacceptable, lacking, and anxious. By putting on a performance, I am avoiding letting anyone get close enough to know the real me, because I am terrified that the real me will have you drop me like a hot potato and move on to someone more friendly, more inviting, more approachable, more easy, more real. I am playing the avoidance game, plain and simple, just covertly and masterfully.

But to add to the complexity, I am also playing the endurance game at the same time. Since I have hammered it into my head that living in the world is unavoidable, the only thing I can do is to face it. So I must grit my teeth and bite my tongue and endure for as long as the illusion lasts.

Neither of these strategies is sustainable. And certainly neither is healthy in the long run. But the fundamental and biggest flaw is this: I shouldn't have to do any of this. If the key to living with Social Anxiety is to learn self-acceptance and realize that there is nothing wrong with me or with being me, the performances are not doing any of that.

In fact it simply reinforces the saddest truth that I have come to realize: I was right. Every performance reinforces the truth that I learned long ago. That I am wrong. That something is wrong with *me*, not with a world that can't accept me.

Every time I slip into a character I am reminded of the fact that I wouldn't have to do this if I was normal. Reminded that I am not normal if I have to go to such extreme lengths just to survive on a day-to-day basis. Reminded of the fact that I wouldn't be accepted for myself, but for a character that I carefully crafted to look like a me I wish I was. Reminded that there is no place in the world for people like me.

Will you forgive me for being the way I am?

Chapter Six
Eat

They started two days ago. The misguided Jiminy Cricket that had led me to this point in the first place was predictably gone, and my own mind was too shot to put two thoughts together and call it a sentence.

My feet were warm. Odd. I was freezing. Everything was cold. But my feet were warm. That was good I guess. Maybe?

Thoughts dripped sluggishly into the swamp pool of my consciousness. Like old honey, the sugared supermarket kind. That didn't say much, thoughts were faded around the edges like old photographs, simultaneously too slow to make out and too fast to understand.

I should really eat.

The piercing pain didn't feel so sharp anymore. Maybe it wasn't so hungry anymore, though why that would be I couldn't even begin to fathom. Who was angry?

Did I eat already?

What?

My lips were dry. I wasn't sure where I was or what day it was, but I knew my lips were dry. Water. Water, please. I pulled my arms under me, elbows bent and ready for the herculean effort to push my body up. It occurred to me I must be lying down. How many classes missed does that make this?

The pressure against my side didn't let up. I hadn't moved. I was certain I had pushed. Did I just push myself on my side or had I always been in this position? Did it matter? I couldn't move.

The shooting pain intensified, a frantic companion to the unwanted realization that I was way too far gone this time, had pushed too far against the limits of a physical body. I was past usefulness. It was quiet.

I tried again. An arm crawled up to my head, jerky and strange like the severed hand of a zombie that's been lopped off. Oh that's my own arm. It looked funny. I saw the moment it lost its pitiful surge of strength and creaked to a halt before it did anything remotely helpful. The ugly green I kept seeing in the background suddenly identified itself as the desk chair. I was facing the room; good I wouldn't have to turn over then.

Move.

Move!

My feet were cold. The thought was at once jarring and confusing and it took a minute to make sense of the fact that I had managed to swing my legs to the ground. Now for the rest of me.

The zombie arm animated again, bent at the wrist and it shook with the effort it took to push my weight up. How much did I weigh now anyway?

I did manage to sit up, but for an odd moment it felt like the room had gotten up with me. It was difficult to distinguish whether the current vision problems were a result of dizziness or if the room was actually blurry around the edges. Was it because of the sunlight? Was it late? What time was it anyway?

Any record of how I managed to stand up and move was not deemed worthy of recalling, but the hand on the mini-fridge door was definitely mine. The fridge was mostly littered with my roommate's energy drinks and her share of sodas. I hadn't been to the store. The last time I went was a memory too far to bother retrieving. There wasn't much in here that was mine. A half empty container of yoghurt, a mandarin that had grown practically senile in solitary confinement in the mini vegetable box. Not a lot to work with.

The futile search bore fruit.

The culinary experiment looked like hash browns. But way too orange to be potato. Carrots? What else was orange? It didn't matter either way, I was far too hungry to care that I didn't like vegetables. I would eat fried tar at this point. Was that why I came to the fridge in the first place? I was certain I had dropped the original reason on the floor somewhere between the bed and the fridge but I was not particularly inclined to go find whatever it was.

The Tupperware cover proved a tougher battle than I anticipated, but it was one I ultimately won. The lumpy irregular contents certainly looked appetizing but the wafting smell was a different army altogether and I lost the battle of keeping my hunger alive. It died like a baby bird fallen out of the nest the second I saw food. The pain, however, was a hardy monster and it made its presence known with a violent spike that had me gasping for breath, hovering awkwardly halfway to the floor.

I grabbed one lumpy whatever-it-was with my bare hand and popped it into my mouth without a second spared for thought. I just needed to appease the beast in my belly. Chew and swallow. Chew and swallow. On my knees before the fridge, I had made it halfway through the hashbrown thing before the oddly amusing thought danced its way to notice: sweet potato. That's what I was eating. Who made a hash brown thing out of sweet potato anyway? It didn't matter, it tasted like ash. Everything tasted like ash. Maybe if it was warm it would have a flavor, but leaving the room to go to the main kitchen was simply out of the question.

Why were my lips so dry?

One more of the cooking experiment followed the first. The pain didn't fade immediately. I knew from experience that it would get sharper first before settling. Soup would have been best, but I was a beggar. And I had long forfeited the right to choose. The nausea that came immediately after was also expected. The gag reflex kicked in before I was ready for it, and I lost the ultimate war. The third sweet potato lump was dropped unceremoniously back in the Tupperware box and the box was thrown into the fridge as if it contained a live grenade. In many ways it did.

I gagged again. The hunger had refused my offering and the aftermath was not going to be pretty. Wherever my roommate was right now, I begged and prayed to a quiet God that she would not come back now.

My stomach heaved again. My arms wrapped around it in vain comfort, tightly trying to hold my diaphragm against the onslaught. I hadn't realized that it was so easy to count ribs, the thought errant and ill-timed.

The food burned in my stomach like acid, furiously protesting the injustice I had done to it by consuming it. It burned and churned and fought. Anyone but me, it screeched. I agreed.

I was at the trashcan just in time for the food to make its enraged reappearance. If it tasted bad going in, it was a million times more unforgiving on its exit. My stomach heaved and heaved till the previous pain was a distant memory and the current burn of agony was my only coherent thought.

I spat out the last of the bile in my mouth, acrid and acidic and bitter as life itself. I should be feeling weaker, but I oddly wasn't. A slight tremble settled into my fingers but little more. The pain was dulled too. Adrenaline probably. Regardless, I wasn't leaving the opportunity to go to waste. The plastic bag that lined the trashcan was tied up, thrown out in the main collection bin in the hall, and replaced with a fresh one in a matter of minutes. The window slid open and the AC turned on full blast got rid of any remaining odors while I brushed it out of my mouth. I avoided the mirror, afraid to look at what it would show me.

I wondered if my roommate would notice if I borrowed one of her sodas. Even if she did, I will buy her another one anyway. The room was back to normal and I was back on the bed, the addition of a stolen soda can in hand, before the shaking set in. It made the can hard to open but practice is a hard passion to beat. The sugar helped pump some energy to my veins even if the gas further burned the abused lining of my insides. I drank slowly this time, relishing the burn with every sip.

I would need to come up with a new game plan. This was too conspicuous.

Sleep came like an uninvited but welcome guest. I wasn't inclined to argue its call, and I was passed out again by the time my friend came back to the room, empty soda can haphazardly placed on the side table.

Chapter Seven
Self-Loathing

I read somewhere once that if you were to see a person with your visage walking toward you on a busy street, you wouldn't recognize your own face. I would kindly like to disagree. I would recognize it instantly. Because I have spent countless hours scrutinizing every excruciating detail of what I look like, spent hours memorizing every imperfection. And imagined putting a fist through it all.

Yes, I handled this topic with the sensitivity of a sledgehammer. Or maybe a wrecking ball. And my evil deed for the day is done. You're singing that song in your head aren't you?

Right, back to the sledgehammer.

I think my issues with my sense of self began when my self-esteem hit zero. And I don't remember a time when it wasn't zero, so I guess it happened pretty early on. So what else is new?

But let's jump right into this very joyful topic, shall we?

It is little secret by now that I am not my biggest fan. I hate the fact that I feel broken. I feel like the presence I am offering the world and the people around me is pointless and burdensome. I feel like a chef who can't cook but insists on having his own restaurant. The very nerve.

I hate the fact that I can't be normal. In any room I enter, I feel like the biggest misfit. A sheep in wolves' clothing.

I hate that I can't turn it off. The feeling that I'm being watched is constantly there. Do you know what anatidaephobia is? It's the fear that somehow, somewhere in the world, a duck is watching you. Not attacking or anything.

Just watching. That's what it feels like for me. That somehow, somewhere, a person is watching me. And judging me of course. Every aspect of my life feels like it's on display.

When I was in high school and college, the feeling was so intense that it felt like my thoughts were on display too. What if someone could read my mind and see just how much filth is filled in it? What if someone was reading my thoughts right now? I tell you, tests were difficult. I couldn't shake the feeling that my thoughts were not private. So I would recite the wrong answers in my head during a quiz, while I wrote down the correct ones. How I managed to pass anything was a miracle in and of itself. See, Mom? There's a reason for the A minuses.

Coming home to my empty apartment as I grew older didn't offer any relief either. For a while I would refuse to turn on the lights at home because I felt like someone was watching. I plastered trash bags to the windows to make sure the neighbors couldn't see me. I should point out at this point that there were no windows opposite my studio room's window. The sad part is in today's world of increasing technological invasiveness, the fear isn't exactly invalid either. But I hate the feeling of vulnerability the fear brings with it. And most of all I hate that I can't fight the feeling despite knowing how irrational the fear is.

I know that it's not exactly a justification for invading someone's privacy, but I hate that even if someone were watching, they wouldn't find anything of value or beauty. Because I hate the way I look and I hate the way I act.

My lack of appreciation for my body began when I was a toddler really. No exaggeration. Like I said. I remember stuff from really long ago.

As a child, I was a chubby baby. My cousins used to smack my chubby little baby tummy and call me 'fatty.' I'm sure they meant it endearingly, but in my head the self-consciousness set in. *I must be really fat*, I thought. And if they are laughing, then that must not be a good thing. I'm ugly.

No one seemed to be contradicting this chain of thought, and so it stuck. All through my childhood as kids laughed and called me fat and pointed at my belly and my chubby pinchable cheeks. All through my adolescence and teenage years as I was surrounded by my classmates. It is an awkward age as it is, and the fact that your body goes on the fritz as you hit puberty doesn't help. I put on weight and God, I hated my slow metabolism. I later learned that this was because of a combination of genetics and a hypothyroid problem, but that didn't make me like my body any better. In fact it just reinforced the notion that it was broken.

As I joined university, I seemed to be surrounded by women with perfect hourglass figures. I, on the other hand, was flat and rectangular. Unless you looked at me from the side; then I looked like the Libra symbol. A rather cruel way to show my star sign in my opinion.

So as soon as I was out of the house and out from under my parents' overprotective wing, I took matters into my own hands. I purposely 'forgot' to eat meals. I cut down my daily intake to a single meal a day. I cut my portion size in half.

The results were stunning. I lost my baby fat in a couple of months. I dropped to a size four in clothing. I actually had a figure. And for the first time in remembrance, I was actually happy with the way I looked.

Now to keep the way my body looked constant, that was a harder battle as any gym-goer would attest to. So I took my methods to the extreme. I started working out, pushing my body to the limits of its endurance until I would be left shaky and pukey. And speaking of pukey, I started to purge. Like I said, I was not afraid to try extreme methods. I half suspect that my ulcer problem was caused by this behavior, but I couldn't care less. The pain in my stomach and the added weight loss simply made me happier. I found it to be a solution for how to keep the weight off. I didn't even need to purposely purge now, it happened all by itself with natural means. But it never seemed enough.

As an adult, and as my conviction in my beliefs matured to something undeniable, people around me started to take notice of my body dysmorphia. I guess it made people uncomfortable when I firmly declared that I was fat and ugly. Especially when all evidence pointed to the contrary. According to my height, my BMI index would indicate that my weight is on the edge of being classified as underweight. That thought scared me. I didn't need an eating disorder diagnosis on top of everything already wrong with me. Now the thing about eating disorders is that you need to be underweight to be diagnosed with most of them. So I changed tactics, all I had to do was keep my weight at this limit and I was golden to keep doing what I was doing.

I did eventually have to get the ulcers checked when I started throwing up blood. Now that the weight loss was no longer happening, the familiar feelings of inadequacy returned. I felt fat and heavy. And I went right back to hating my body.

That is until I lost my Chancellor's List scholarship and award. Especially because I lost it by 0.02 points on my cumulative GPA. Such a narrow margin coupled with the fact that I knew I lost it because I couldn't suck up to my design professor the way she liked it drove me over the edge. I was burning with pent-up anger that had nowhere to go. It was undirected and raw and so I turned it to the one thing I believed not only warranted my anger for failing to meet my lofty expectations but also was able to take the weight of my fury without judgment. Myself. I began to self-harm.

Now, I should clarify, I had been engaging in some manner of self-destructive behavior since I was eleven. I would use a pin or my nails to scratch my skin. It worked because not only can 'accidents' that look like a scratch happen in everyday life, but the scars would not remain with so shallow a scratch. It helped matters that I was naturally clumsy so explaining away the marks was easy. Only problem was no one was asking me anything. This was when invisibility had its perks and challenges. I was so invisible that no one was even noticing my cry for help.

Over time, a scratch or two was not enough. I would cover a whole limb in the thin red lines till the skin stung with the sharp pain. And the itching would drive me crazy as they healed. But the next day, the pain would be gone and I would have to redo it all over again on another limb. It's not like anyone was asking why I was limping or scratching, but still I was careful to only mark the body parts no one would accidentally see.

Pain became a crutch. A reminder that I was alive in the numbness I was drowning in. Pain felt welcome, a relief from the failure that was me.

In university, the night of the Award ceremony, two things changed. I upgraded from pins to blades and I cut for the first time. I mean I was in interior design, surrounded by art knives and blades of so many different kinds; it's as if God himself had given me the tools for my grim task. And second, it was the first time I self-harmed in anger.

All the anger poured out on the one person responsible for my misery: Me. All the hatred boiled forth like the blood from the wound and I admit I nearly passed out from the shock of the endorphin rush and the sheer release. For once, my head was quiet.

The pain lasted for days as the deep wound healed slowly. It felt like I was finally getting the pain and punishment I deserved for being a lowly worm that I was. Self-harm out of anger quickly became my new release. It felt justified. The pain felt like I was finally getting the punishment I deserved for being the broken thing that I was. It was punishment for daring to dream of things I could never hope to achieve.

And in a messed up way, it made me feel better. That was expected. What was unexpected was the other side-effect of my brutal self-harm. I began to like my body again. The more scars I got the better I felt.

It felt like all the pain I carried so invisibly and discreetly in my head was manifested. The scars proved it was real, that I was not crazy. Well, completely crazy anyway. The condition that made me hate myself had met its remedy. I was reborn in blood and blade silver.

In fact, I actually began to take care of my body. Have you heard the fitness mantra that if you take care of your body your body will take care of you? I actually began to believe it. Only if I took care of my body and let it heal and let it grow healthy, could it serve me well by letting me rip it apart over and over and over. And so I pampered it.

I started exercising again. But this time like a sane person. I took up dancing in the privacy of my room. I bought lotions and potions. I ate healthy. In no time my haggard body began to look better. My skin cleared up. I glowed. My stamina improved. I felt healthy. And I felt beautiful for the first time. Not because of the glowing or anything so mundane. My scars made me beautiful.

The more I covered myself in them, the more beautiful I felt and the better I treated my body. It was as if I was given a reason to take care of it. I rather enjoyed playing nurse to the bleeding oozing wounds as I carefully sanitized the wound and wrapped it up to keep infection away. I rather enjoyed the peaceful deep sleep afterward. I enjoyed the meal I would reward myself with for being a good girl and taking the pain so well. Life became about punishment and reward. Both administered by me.

I realize how unhealthy this sounds. I was basically beating myself up when I got angry and then treating myself to say sorry. I was essentially in an abusive relationship with myself. And I liked it. Does that make me kinky?

Eventually I started doing patterns with the cuts. Bands and swirls. If this is going to stay on my body forever, it might as well be beautiful, as macabre as that sounds.

I read a blog once that if you self-harm, know that you are marking your body forever. This is how you will look on your wedding day. It is what you will look like when you have kids and they ask you what is that on your body. Well, it's a very good thing I don't intend to get married or have kids. Who could ever love me the way I love myself?

Nobody.

I'm fine with that. I can learn to be fine with that as long as I have my scars.

Chapter Eight
Narcissist

When I was young and easily impressionable, I used to watch Supernatural. I'm about to lose a bunch of readers aren't I?

I didn't start watching it for the plot. I didn't know at the time that the first five seasons were amazingly done. Credit where it is due. In fact, I didn't even start watching it 'cause of all the pretty. And let's be real, Jared and Jensen are really, really perty. No, I started watching a horror show because I was a chicken. Counterintuitive you say? Welcome to my life.

I hated horror movies as a child. Put on something scary and I would refuse to go to the bathroom because I'd be too afraid to be on my own for even a second for fear that some demon or ill-formed ghost would scare the living shit out of me. Nighttime was the worst.

As I grew older, this scaredy behavior became a source of shame for me. I was embarrassed of myself for being such a fraidy cat. Something needed to change. So I decided the best thing to do was to face my fear. All I needed to do was wait till something scary came on TV and then I would watch it and bite my terror in the ass once and for all.

In those days, we lived in Niger. So I wasn't exactly going to get some great internet service that I could stream the show online. No, I had to watch it the old fashioned way: on TV. And all that was playing at the time was season one of Supernatural, the scariest season in my opinion.

I do admit I spent quite a few episodes hiding behind my mother squealing at her to tell me when the ghost was off-screen. She got more mirth out of this than anyone as she would purposely lie and tell me it's gone and like a naive child who trusts their mother with their very sanity I would peer out only to find that the ghost was ghosting it up and whew. I'm not bitter.

But I do owe it to her, because watching the show did eventually diminish my fear of the horror genre. I can now watch any horror movie and be fine…after a day or two that is. Except 'It.' I refuse to watch It. Clowns. Creepy.

And to top it off, I did get into the show. And develop a massive crush on Jared Padalecki as Sam. Yeah OK, go ahead and laugh but I have a thing for the cute nerd, OK?

So when Jared announced that he was struggling with depression and anxiety, I felt a little connected to him. And when he launched his Always Keep Fighting campaign, I was amongst the first to jump on board. I was so happy that finally mental health was getting the respect and recognition it deserved. I hoped that slowly the stigma surrounding mental illnesses would ease away, like my fear of horror movies.

What I did not expect was the way I would react to the growing movement of AKF. The more people found the courage to voice their struggles and find companionship with others like themselves, the more disillusioned I became.

Something felt wrong. Everybody in the world seemed to be struggling with some kind of mental disorder. I know everybody in the world has a struggle, something they have to fight through. But this felt…different. And I found myself becoming apathetic to the growing movement, and then downright resentful.

How could this be possible? What happened to the numbers that only a small percentage of the population suffered the way I did? Or maybe that was just part of the stigma and stereotype that the only people who deserved to be called mentally ill and struggling were the ones who had had some traumatic experience happen to them. Something that warranted their struggle and allowed them to call themselves mentally ill. And the more stories I heard the more it seemed true. And the more I hated myself for not having such a story. By what right could I call myself mentally ill? What was my struggle anyway? Why did I deserve the title of having a mental disorder when I felt I hadn't earned it?

I guess that was the problem all along. The problem was with me, not with people who I started to believe called themselves mentally ill for the attention and sympathy it would grant them.

I was mentally ill; I had a struggle that I faced every day. Where was my sympathy? Granted it was an incorrect expectation, but I did expect people to understand what it meant when I was telling them that I suffered from Social Anxiety. I expected people to back off from crowding my space with their everyday demands to be part of society. I expected the pressure and strain I felt every day to ease off slightly. I saw that happen to other people. I saw others being excused because "they were a special case." It just didn't seem to be happening to me.

Granted part of it was my fault. A funny thing about social anxiety is that it fosters the belief that nobody should know that you have Social Anxiety. It's like Fight Club. First rule of Fight Club is that there is no Fight Club. Because Social Anxiety harbors the belief that if anyone knew about the condition, it would open the door for judgment. I couldn't handle that. So I kept my condition secret and protected it with my life.

But the need for sympathy is strong and a powerful force to deny. As human beings, we just want to be understood and accepted for who we are. And I felt that need keenly. Being unable to say it outright, I took to dropping hints. I would allow myself to stutter when trying to order food, or show signs of panic in classes or presentations, or refuse to talk and interact at dinner parties. I thought I was making it pretty obvious. But no one seemed to take notice. I just couldn't seem to catch the break I so desperately thought I deserved and that I so longingly wanted.

And I began to wonder; was there something wrong with me? Was I being and acting like an attention-seeker? Was I being a hypocrite? The fear of that being true ruminated in my mind, a slow steady poison as I learned to hate both myself for wanting sympathy from others and the world for denying it to me.

Then sometime later I made a friend at work. She was only here on a temporary contract, but something about us just clicked. She was struggling with extreme mood swings and depression and suicidal tendencies. And I felt like if anyone could, she could understand me. And to her credit, she did.

She got my sense of humor, as hers was just as dark and self-deprecating. She got my panic attacks as she had them too. She hated the presence of people just as much as I did. We fit like two peas in a sick pod.

But then I realized something as I talked her through a panic attack in the office toilet for the second time that week. She couldn't help me.

I wanted someone to help me. I wanted someone to listen to me. I wanted someone to *try* to understand me and fail. I couldn't handle someone telling me they understood me because I didn't believe they did at all. How could anyone understand what my life feels like? How could anyone understand the way I have to pretend to be someone else just to get by? How could anyone understand the hunger of three days without food because you're just so terrified to pick up the phone or go out to get a meal? How could anyone possibly understand the way I felt about my scars?

I wanted to feel special. I wanted someone to tell me I was special because I lived with this debilitating condition so well. I wanted someone to wholeheartedly try to understand me even when they know they never will completely. Was I a narcissist? Was something wrong with me?

All I knew was that to understand me and help me is a full-time job. I wanted it to be a full-time job. I wanted someone to focus on me the way Gabriel Iglesias focuses on a taco. And I wasn't going to get that from my friend. She had her own hurdles to climb. She could never focus on helping me.

Neither could anyone else. If everyone has some sort of struggle that they are fighting, who could help me fight mine?

If everyone is so busy fighting their own battles, what companionship could they offer anyone else?

"You are not alone," the AKF campaign promises. "There are others out there like you."

Yes. True. Too many people like me, in fact. But how does that help me? They are too busy trying to keep their own shit and sanity together. At the end of the day, I am actually very much alone. My fight will be my fight and my fight alone. No one can help me. No one is in the position to give me what I want or what I need.

That thought makes me feel very much alone. And very very stupid. I want to be the center of someone's world like the little narcissist that I am. Is that really so wrong? Having spent my whole life in the shadows, is it really so wrong of me to crave a little light?

Now I know what you are thinking; it sounds like somebody needs a boyfriend. Ha, ha. Find me someone who can put up with me and I'll consider it.

But you want to know what the real tragedy is? I want something I cannot have. I crave light, but I cannot handle being seen. I want to be the center of someone's world, but I cannot handle being the center of anything, never mind that what I am asking for is unreasonable.

What is wrong with me?

Chapter Nine
Therapy

I never imagined myself doing therapy. No one does I guess. It's not exactly up there in the bucket list of things to do.

I suppose my therapy technically started when I was still in high school when my mother reported to my homeroom teacher that she was concerned about my behavior. I never heard of it again so I suppose that never amounted to much.

I did actually try in college. Before I was reported by the concerned professor, I paid a visit to the counselor's office of my own accord. I went in and awkwardly declared that I think I was struggling with depression and suicidal thoughts when the bored receptionist asked me why I thought I needed counseling. The receptionist then proceeded to sigh, actually sigh, and clicked a few times on her computer before she morosely asked what time I would prefer. I asked for a slot two days from then as I figured that should give me some time to mentally prepare myself but not enough to overthink and chicken out. The woman nodded and then proceeded to ignore me.

Was I done? Was that it?

I stood around awkwardly waiting for her to say something else but she seemed happy enough to ignore my entire existence and stare dejectedly at the computer. So I left, entirely put off by her attitude. Later that evening I received an email from the counselor services that my appointment had been cancelled. I took that as a sign from God that this was a bad idea and dropped the thought of seeing the counselor at all. It was a semester after that that I received the email that I *had to* see the counselor.

At first I ignored that email, the distaste of my first visit still fresh in my mind. I ignored the second one too. But when the third one declared that it was mandatory since a professor had reported me, I feared the repercussions if the university decided to get in touch with my parents. Up until this point, my parents had never mentioned anything abnormal about me other than the shyness so I was happy to continue living under the belief and knowledge that they knew nothing of what I was struggling with.

So begrudgingly, I went to the counselor for a second time.

This time there was no receptionist to hurdle. I simply announced that I was told to come here and ten minutes later I was being shown into a stuffy little office stacked high with papers. The room was cold.

The doctor seated at the desk seemed friendly enough but I was not about to forgive her for making me come here against my will. And so I refused to cooperate.

"Hello, can you tell me your name, please?" she asked while ruffling through some files.

I didn't answer and chose to stare at the clock instead of her face. For once in my life, I didn't care what she thought of me. I was angry and I wanted her to know it. When she didn't get a reply, she finally stopped scrabbling and looked up, her glasses balanced precariously on her nose. She was desi. And I immediately didn't trust her; Desis have a hard time looking past a destructive culture but insist it must be followed to a T.

The doctor repeated her question and I again ignored it. This time I gave her a pointed stare from the corner of my eye to let her know I meant business. She got the message and turned to her computer instead. "Hafsa?" she asked after checking whatever it was she checked.

I blinked.

"Can you tell me why you're here, Hafsa?"

I balked. If she had to ask me that after making me come here, then this was going to go nowhere. It was also not winning her any points in my book.

I crossed my arms and went back to staring at the clock.

"Can you tell me which major you're in?"

If you bothered to look up my name from your system, shouldn't it also give you that information?

The doctor tried asking a few more questions about me, about my parents, whether I had any friends, if I was enjoying my classes. But I was immoveable. I refused to indulge her. I was here to say I fulfilled my obligation, now fuck off.

To her credit, she kept trying. "Do you feel lost, Hafsa?"

Shit, yes. But I'm not telling you that.

The doctor sighed. Finally, she told me that if I didn't cooperate she would have to tell my parents and professors that I was unfit and needed therapy sessions. That worked. That scared me. I shuffled nervously and looked her in the face for as long as I could before dropping my gaze back to the floor.

"Do you want that?" she asked.

I shook my head no, still staring at the floor.

"OK. I'm going to give you some forms to fill out. Can you do that?"

I considered refusing for a minute but her threat still hung heavy in the air, so I nodded once.

She passed a stack of form towards me and gave me a pen and told me to begin.

So begin I did. I put the stack on my lap and filled out the forms. There was a self-esteem scale. There were several anxiety ones. There were several depression ones. And a few others that I was definitely sure were not relevant. I guess because I was not cooperating with her she was keeping all her bases covered. Just in case. It took me fifteen minutes but I finally had all the forms answered.

She smiled at me encouragingly and I wrestled with the urge to hold on to my anger and not smile back. I was failing so I looked away.

The doctor started tallying up the results from the forms and my heart sank as I watched her. I was on the extreme side of the spectrum in almost every category, form after form. It took her ten minutes of silent work where she hmm'd and mhm'd to herself. By the time she finally looked up at me, my heart had sunk into my stomach.

Don't say I'm crazy. Don't say I'm crazy. Just tell me what's wrong with me but don't say I'm crazy.

"OK, Hafsa. It looks like you're struggling with some pretty severe depression and some worrying anxiety levels."

Heh. 'Worrying anxiety.' This woman was a genius. Heh.

Then she put the forms down and leaned forward on her desk and began in a very serious tone. "Hafsa, do you know what is Social Anxiety?"

I didn't. I saw it on some of the forms but that was it. I had a bad feeling about this and where it was going.

"Do you ever think of how people think of you? Do you find yourself concerned about how you look, how you walk, how you talk?"

Only all the time, lady.

I nodded apprehensively.

"How do you feel about speaking in public?"

I couldn't shake my head fast enough.

"OK, do you find yourself concerned about what your professors or your classmates think of you?"

I nodded.

"What about your friends?"

I nodded again.

Shit.

"OK, Hafsa. I think you may have Social Anxiety Disorder…"

She kept talking about some more tests and some questions and whether I would be OK with coming back here again or seeing a specialized therapist, but I wasn't listening anymore. The word disorder kept ringing in my head like a death knell.

I'm crazy. I'm crazy. I'm crazy. I'm crazy.

Anything but that. Not in our culture, not in my family. It couldn't be possible. I could never show my face again.

I don't know when I left the doctor's office, but I found myself walking back to the dorms in a daze, convinced that if I pushed against the revelation hard enough it would go away.

I got to the dorms and immediately pulled open my laptop to google 'social anxiety disorder.' And everything I read fit me like a tailor-made glove. It was like I was reading my life on the screen. And the more I read, the more I was filled with dread. I was going to have to face the facts; it looked like I had Social Anxiety Disorder.

I finally had a name to my madness.

And the thought terrified me.

I never spoke or thought of the counselor's death sentence again. I buried it deep down and kept on doing what I was doing: digging a hole and burying myself deeper and deeper and deeper. Until I hit rock bottom again.

Weirdly, the visit to the counselor helped put things into perspective for me. I was slowly ruining myself and it wasn't going to do any good. I was not letting something like insanity control me. Hell no. I was going to prove it wrong and show it that I could do what needed to be done. That worked for a couple years. I got through my masters, got my first job. And then the routine hit me with the force of a planetoid and I was sent reeling. Doing the same thing every day, all day. It was tedious and it was hard and I was not equipped to handle the very real-world consequences of meetings and presentations. When I landed my current job, the feelings increased tenfold. Talking to peers and making decisions and phone calls and talking to consultants and attending meetings and on and on and on. I couldn't do it. The phone rang and my heart stopped. Boss called me to her office and I nearly wet myself. Someone asked me a question in a meeting and I nearly launched into a panic attack.

It had to stop.

The anxiety multiplied and the depression I was barely holding at bay crashed over me once again. When I finally ran out of real estate on my body to put more scars on to make me feel better, I decided it was time to get help. For real this time.

It was an older, much more desperate, much more heavily scarred, much more scared young woman who went around Sharjah looking for a therapist.

Looking for a therapist turns out to be half the struggle of therapy itself it would seem. First of all, everyone was in Dubai and since I didn't own a car that was simply not going to be feasible. There were a grand total of four options in Sharjah. Now finding someone among those options who was specialized in social anxiety was a challenge. So I read through their profiles until I narrowed down on one Dr. Marie who proclaimed her interest in the disorder.

I loitered around the idea for several days trying to work up the nerve to make an appointment. Luckily there was an option for an online appointment, effectively sparing me the torture of making a phone call. So before I could talk myself out of the idea, I went for it.

I regretted it.

From the first day, I didn't feel like we clicked. She was abrupt and to the point and had a loud voice for a small lady. She felt like a scouring sponge. Sure it will get the job done, but it didn't mean the dish was going to like any second of the cleaning process. Me, on the other hand, I was a non-stick. Meaning scouring sponges and I don't really get along very well.

From our very first meeting, she developed her own idea of what I was struggling with and it didn't seem to be the Social Anxiety that was far up on the list of priorities. She seemed taken with the idea of my self-harm, and the Social Anxiety was just an annoying gnat that was getting in the way. I felt it was the very opposite. I didn't want to tell her my counselor experience in college in detail, because she seemed to be one of those people who either jumped on the bandwagon or burned it down.

Marie made me take several tests again, some of which I recognized. Everyone seemed to be taking the same test off the same website it seemed. But when I was done, she was convinced I had Borderline Personality Disorder. Granted, I scored extremely high on that test (what can I do? I'm an overachiever) but I didn't feel like it was the cause of the Social Anxiety. If I even had B.P.D., it was probably as a by-product of having S.A.D. for so long. But when I tried to tell her that, I was rather harshly reminded of the fact that she was the one with a license in psychology, not me. And being me, I let the matter simmer on the backburner rather than try to voice my thoughts again.

Another thing that Marie was excessively focused on was the fact that at that point I didn't seem to be eating. That was true. When I went to see her, I was so nervous I hadn't eaten for three days in fear of the nausea that bubbled up whenever I got anxious. If I hadn't eaten, there would be nothing to throw up, right? Mostly wrong, but OK. I admit, her concern was validated. I didn't believe it when people told me, but I knew I was thin for my height. I was barely keeping within the weight limit I had set for myself. She gave me her number and told me to tell her when I ate that evening. I didn't eat. And I certainly didn't tell her.

When I went to my next appointment, that was the first question she asked me. Had I eaten?

I lied and said yes so she would let the matter drop. It made me uncomfortable. I hadn't eaten since the day before as I was on a quest to really discuss the therapy methods she planned to use. I wanted to discuss my Social Anxiety Disorder with her but she beat me to the punch.

"Have you cut recently?" she asked.

I considered lying and saying no, but figured that wouldn't do me any good. So I told the truth and nodded.

"Why?" she asked.

"Because I had a fight with my friend." That wasn't true. It had never escalated to a fight. My friend had simply told me she was going to come see me, and then hadn't. I had felt betrayed, betrayal had led to anger, anger had led to guilt, and guilt had led to punishment and Bob's your uncle. It was stupid to say the least.

"Tell me about it," Marie demanded.

So I made up a story as close to the truth as I could manage.

"See? That's a sign of borderline disorder." She seemed so sure. Fine, let's say it was true, that wasn't why I had come to her for help. I didn't intend to stop cutting. What I intended to do was overcome my worthless existence and become a contributing member to the social circle around me. So this was my chance.

"Can we focus on the Social Anxiety?" I quietly asked.

"Yeah, we'll work on that but that's not a real problem."

I stared at her. That wasn't true at all. So I told her how I couldn't handle crowded places, told her how I couldn't order food, how I couldn't leave the house, how I felt ashamed of the person I was, how I felt I couldn't be myself in front of my friends and family much less my coworkers and strangers, how I couldn't turn on the lights at home.

And to prove me wrong, she suggested a simple test. Go to the elevator, get in, ride to the top floor and come back.

And I blanched. I couldn't do it. The very thought sent my skin prickling and itching and tightened my chest. I shook my head emphatically no. I couldn't do it. Not in a crowded hospital elevator.

But she was adamant. So was I.

Till she declared she was coming with me, and I didn't have an answer to that. So I gave in. And thus the ill-fated elevator test was conducted, and failed. I had won, I had proven my point. Yay me.

Back in the relative unsafety of her office she demanded I stop crying. *Yeah sure, lady, like I can control it.*

"If it's that severe, how do you live?" she finally asked with a voice layered with pity and judgment.

"I don't," I sniffled. *That was the whole point I was here, weren't you listening?*

"You need medication. Have you considered taking medication for your anxiety?"

I had. And I desperately wanted to but culture got in the way. My parents were firmly against the idea of taking medications for mental illnesses. They claimed they were full of side-effects and did nothing useful and they rejected the idea with such vehemence that I was scared to even bring it up.

"See this doctor tomorrow," Marie said, writing down a name.

And then deciding I had had enough for that day, she dismissed me and I shot home like the hounds of hell were after me.

The next day, I made an appointment (online) with the psychiatrist she had recommended. He was in Dubai but when I voiced my timid question for how often I had to see him, he said only once a month. I could do that.

He decided he would have to conduct his own diagnosis. For the third time, I was asked the same questions about how long I had struggled with depression, how long with anxiety, what I did to feel better. And once again I recounted the self-harm, the feeling of being watched, the inability to turn it all off. Once again, I filled out the same forms (seriously, what is this website, I might as well print out and fill a bunch of copies to save everyone some time).

He concluded that I definitely had a social phobia, as well as Borderline and Obsessive Compulsive Disorder and Generalized Anxiety. OK, the Generalized Anxiety I could sort of understand but O.C.D.? Buddy, have you seen the state of my apartment? Ain't no way I have O.C.D. I'm one of those leave-it-where-it-fell type people. Not that that's a real indicator or O.C.D., but my point is I am not compulsive or obsessive.

He prescribed an antidepressant and an anti-anxiety medication and told me I was good to go. I didn't tell my parents I had started medication.

A week passed, nothing happened. Another week, and I felt remarkably worse. The depression had been poked like one pokes a bear. I had made it angry and it was not happy. I told the psychiatrist about this and he said it was normal and to just give it another month. I told Marie and she too told me to wait.

Once more I opened my laptop and googled what to do if your therapist doesn't listen to you. Most of the advice said to talk to the therapist and clarify your goals for what therapy is supposed to do for you. Yeah, that sounded like a lot of talking and opening yourself up to a lot of judgment and I have Social Anxiety don't you know.

But there didn't seem to be another way around it so I decided to add my own 'Hiccup flair' to the advice. I wrote a letter detailing how I felt like my input wasn't being considered and that I wanted to focus on the things I felt were important to me at the current time. The next session I sat through the same routine of the questions about whether I had eaten, or whether I had cut, whether I had been to the grocery store like Marie had asked me to. She spent the hour discussing my "fight" with my friend again. All the while I waited for my chance to give her the letter. Finally the end of the session came about and without a word I left her office.

This wasn't right. If I was going to invest my time and money into therapy then I needed to communicate. Which meant I had to give Marie that letter.

Easier said than done. My hands started to shake and I realized I was having difficulty swallowing. But resolutely I opened my purse, snuck into her office again like a weasel, deposited the piece of paper on her desk, and slunk out like the slimy piece of shit that I was.

I regretted the decision instantly and I wondered if there was a way to sneak back inside and get the letter before she read it.

No! Enough! I did the right thing!

And with that I left, trying to hold my head high.

Whether the letter did anything good is still up for debate though at this point in time I would have to say yes, it did. Two days later I received a text from Marie simply declaring that she thought I should see another therapist. It was followed by another text that read she could help, but only if her clients trusted her. Followed by a smiley face. A fucking smiley face.

What the hell?

Trust? Isn't trust earned slowly over time? What sort of counterintuitive method was this where you blindly trust someone to poke around in your head without a say in the matter? I felt sorry for her patients. Now, I am glad I sent that cursed letter, but at the time, drugged up on an antidepressant that wasn't suiting me and feeling like the world was coming to an end, the text crushed me. I felt like my own therapist had given up on me and dumped me via text message no less. I felt like I was a hopeless case, broken beyond repair if even a professional refused to see me. All I could do for the umpteenth time was to cry my heart out in despair.

It was a few weeks before I got the nerve to try again with therapy. The drugs I was still taking were making me feel like shit and I needed help. So once again I got to searching for help. This time I didn't care for psychologists. I just needed a psychiatrist to fix me. I found a little specialist psychiatric clinic in Sharjah and with all my last hopes pinned on it, I actually picked up the phone to call for an appointment. These guys didn't have online appointments. Not a great sign.

When I called, a nurse told me that there were no appointments; that you just come between 5 P.M. and 9 P.M. and it was first come first serve. Even more of a not-so-great sign.

When I got out of the taxi to see an old-looking apartment building in the desi part of Sharjah, my heart sank. This looked like one of those places where you have a 'bank' in a rented apartment building. The elevator crawled up to the fifth floor and sure enough the psychiatric clinic was across from a 'Canara Bank.' Not a great sign.

The place looked shady: No card reader, airplane seats for the waiting area, dim lighting.

The nurses were really friendly, however, and with practiced ease, registered my ID and told me to wait for my turn. After a twenty minute wait, my name was called and a nurse took me into a little room to check my vitals. "Good," she said looking at my weight on the scale. I felt a small modicum of relief that my diet plan was working.

Another twenty minutes and I was called to go to room number three for Dr. Brian. I gave a piddly little embarrassing knock and entered when I was told to come in. A desi man sat behind a laptop at his desk, dignified and with a demeanor that invited conversation. His pepper hair made him look distinguished, along with the button-up shirt and slacks that he wore. Little eyeglasses perched delicately on a rather soft-looking nose.

He listened patiently to my misadventures, interjecting with a question where I blabbered or was unclear. Immediately, I took to him. This was what a doctor should be like. Overcome with relief and renewed hope, I started to cry again. Yeah, I know. I do that a lot.

"You've suffered a lot it seems," he observed. Very astute observation, Doc. He definitely got it.

I sniffled, not knowing how to respond to that. But it seemed I didn't have to. He prescribed me a different antidepressant, the same anti-anxiety meds, and told me to come back in two weeks. I wanted to tell him that I didn't think the anti-anxiety pills were working; all they did was make me astoundingly sleepy and it was getting me in trouble at work. But I didn't have the courage to do that so I let it go. Like I always did.

Two weeks saw no improvement, so he added an antipsychotic to help speed things up. I wasn't sure how I felt about that, but I was grateful he did something rather than simply tell me to wait. Two more weeks actually saw improvement. Finally I didn't feel like roadkill. I saw joy in life. I wanted to do things. See things. I wanted to travel! I wanted to take singing courses like I'd always wanted. Life was full of opportunity.

I took a trip to Sweden. I went aurora-hunting. I rode in a dog-sled. I took a road trip with my friends.

And a couple months in, I was inexplicably drawn back into the deep dark pit from whence I had just climbed. It was as if my happiness had scorned the force of my depression and it kicked me in the teeth. I was back to being sad and empty.

I couldn't understand it; I was doing everything right. How? Why?

We upped the dosage and a few weeks later the problem fixed itself. Only to repeat a couple months later. We upped the dosage again, the problem fixed itself again, and reappeared in a couple months again.

The pattern became a cause for worry as far as I was concerned. I was on medication, by all rights this shouldn't be happening. Having grown comfortable with Dr. Brian, I was able to part-ways raise my concern to him and he mentioned we might have to keep a lookout for bipolar. Yeah add that to the list of everything wrong with me. Periodic lapses of worsening depression followed by periods of happiness. But the problem was, I didn't show the symptom of mania, a key component of bipolar disorder. Overall, he didn't seem too concerned and declared that if we needed to change the dosage or the antidepressant again, then that's what we will do.

You guessed it. The answer did not please me or reassure me in any way. That was by no means a sustainable solution. And more importantly it didn't address the problem of why the depressive episodes were recurring with such regularity. Google turned out to be my best friend again as I furiously looked up Bipolar Disorder and whether I may have it or not.

As it turns out, there were two types of Bipolar Disorder. Type I was the well-known cycle of extreme depression and mania. And then there was Type II, the lesser known and lesser studied. Probably because it wasn't as glamourous as the first type. While it had the extreme depressive episodes, the non-depressive parts of the cycle were less severe forms of mania, called hypomania. Essentially, this translates to a period of heightened mood and a symptom-free state of euthymia. If I did indeed have bipolar disorder, this type II sounded like the best candidate. Especially considering the first thing I did when I was in a good mood was book a trip somewhere. Which is a feat with a Pakistani passport mind you. So far I had taken an impromptu trip to Georgia and another to London. Both were a definite strain on my bank account and were a decision I regretted making when the high wore off. It was definitely something worth discussing, in my opinion. The question now was how to bring it up again in our next session without making the doctor think I didn't trust his judgment or his hopefully up-to-date knowledge of the Diagnostic and Statistical Manual of Mental Disorders. Not only was I still sore from the Marie fiasco, but I feared Dr. Brian's judgment if he thought I was self-diagnosing through Google.

So I let the matter drop as my mood improved again and waited for the next depressive episode.

A few months into seeing Dr. Brian, we decided I should start therapy and conduct a proper psychometric personality test. I found the thought quite funny. Wasn't an analysis the first step, not the middle step? But deciding it wasn't worth the bother to bring that up, I submitted to having my mind probed again. I was introduced to Dr. Sameer, the clinical psychologist, and was once again subjected to the same line of questioning beginning with the ever-present opening tagline: "Tell me why you're here." Shrinks really need to come up with a better opening statement. This one gets old fast.

The psychometric test turned out to be a reintroduction to my old friends, the forms. I was tempted to fill them in from memory, but I refrained and chose to fill them in the old-fashioned way as honestly as I could. Once again I was told that I most definitely had Social Anxiety Disorder. Which was great, imagine if we had been treating the wrong thing all these months.

I didn't have high hopes of ever getting treated at this point, but Dr. Sameer was confident that there was a cure. I didn't believe him, but I didn't tell him that and let him run his Cognitive Behavioral Therapy experiment on me. And thus began my misadventures with counseling.

We began with exercises to expose me to the concept of speaking in public. Dr. Sameer would give me topics that I would have to present to him in a ten-minute talk. I admit I did not see the point of the exercise at all. I knew how to present. I knew all the bells and whistles and tips and tricks. The trick I needed to learn was how to believe in myself. Exposure wasn't going to help, I had been exposed enough. What I needed were the tools to manage the overwhelming anxiety. Admittedly, the first presentation was awkward and bumpy and Dr. Sameer was kind enough to point out my flaws, not yet familiar with the fact that I was an overly sensitive bitch and did not know how to take constructive criticism with grace. I didn't want to do this exercise but I figured it might just be faster to pass this part of the therapy using my repertoire of public speaking skills. I ace-d the next presentation, and blew the one after that out of the water. I was flawless. I was even proud of myself for once. But life has a way of throwing a wrench in the path of your progress. The next presentation was given in the presence of one of the nurses in the clinic. I immediately lost my confidence. The presentation was shaky but I managed to pull through till the end before I succumbed to the panic attack that had been building and was reduced to a shuddering wheezing mess.

To remedy the situation, Dr. Sameer tried to prove to me that everyone faced anxiety when presenting or speaking in public. Nobody was perfect. Problem was, I couldn't care less. People I could forgive. Forgive myself, I could not. I shocked myself with the utter apathy with which I regarded other people's fear. All I wanted to do was cure my own. It didn't matter to me that other people messed up too; what I needed to do was be absolutely *perfect* because if I wasn't people would *judge* me, couldn't anybody understand that?

But how could cowardly little me ever voice so horrible a thought? Easy. I didn't. I pretended to play along just to get this part of the therapy over with. The next step in my therapy plan devastated me.

Dr. Sameer suggested that I study the way people around me interacted with each other. I inwardly rolled my eyes at the assignment; again, I knew the conversation techniques. What I lacked was the confidence to engage those skills.

But like the diligent little student that I am, observe I did. I observed people in the waiting room saunter up and ask for the Wifi password. Something I could never do 'cause I feared the "kids these days with their wifi, what a waste of youth." I watched women buy sanitary pads and cat food and diet yoghurt at the same time and approach the cashier in the grocery store with no sense of embarrassment whatsoever. Something I could never do 'cause of "oh we've got a PMSing crazy cat lady over here." I watched my friend order a large salted caramel latte with no apprehension whatsoever. Something I couldn't do 'cause "Large eh? You better have a great gym membership, sweetheart." I watched my coworkers interject their opinions in meetings, utterly self-assured in what they were saying. Something I couldn't even dream of doing 'cause "you gotta earn your right to have your opinion heard."

Everyone around me, stranger or not, was fearless. Nobody seemed to care about what someone might think of them. All that mattered was what they needed in that moment and nothing more. Everyone seemed utterly sure of the fact that they deserved whatever they were asking for. It was so easy for them when even the simplest thing was impossibly difficult for me. I could never be that carefree, that self-confident, that sure. And the realization broke me. I felt more trapped than ever. It was like there was a thick glass between me and the world. I felt cut off and hopeless. Any optimistic promise of a cure was a lie, or naive. Nobody fully understood the utter seclusion that Social Anxiety cursed me to endure. Not even the people trying to help me.

Any progress that I had made was washed away. And Dr. Brian suggested that we stop therapy immediately. It obviously wasn't working for me. Even the holy grail of cognitive behavioral therapy had failed me.

"You're a very unique person," Dr. Brian told me, trying to make me feel better. Understatement of the year. And I believe the word you are looking for is 'hopeless,' Doc.

"You've suffered enough," he declared sympathetically as he upped my dosage once again.

Chapter Ten
Panic

I peeked out from under my comforter, a quick glance to make sure I was alone. I wasn't. My roommate was standing by the wardrobes putting the finishing touches to her appearance. A jacket here, add a pair of boots there, and she was on her way to becoming another version of her carefully crafted self.

It occurred to me, not for the first time, that we could not have been more polarized. Whilst I hid my frame behind oversized sweaters, hoodies, and jackets, my roommate knew exactly how to accent hers. Her demeanor and the way she carried herself was advertisement enough that this was a person confident within the confines of their own skin. Whether she was aware of the fact that she often looked like a page out of a clothing catalogue was often the subject of my personal debates. Watching my roommate casually wrap a silk scarf as a neckerchief had me a firm believer that she knew exactly what she was doing with her appearance, even if she was not aware of the oodles of envious looks she received behind her back.

The only similarity we seemed to share in common was the odd preference for dark colors. I liked dark colors because they provided a blanket of comfort, an invisible shield that had people second-guessing whether they really wanted to approach me or not. My roommate seemed to simply like dark colors. A sneaking suspicion voiced that perhaps it matched the dark edges of her personality but it was dismissed as objectively unfair. I didn't know anything about my roommate, much less have the right to judge her.

It had been a month after all and we had yet to know each other's names, a most awkward predicament. It was little secret that she was a constant source of terror for me, a fact I am certain she knew. So whether she backed off from consideration or simply dismissal of the odd creature that I am, it was beyond my ability to answer. It was not from lack of trying; she had tried to ask several times in the first week or so of her arrival, but my own inability to answer due to the treacherous snake that choked me every time I opened my mouth to respond was the main culprit. How odd I must have looked to her. A more honest answer would be rude, and it would be justly fair for her to make that assumption about me. I had tried to employ my powers of observation to discern her identity, but being too afraid to approach her or the dorm supervisor for answers and too cowardly to dig through her belongings to find a name, dead end was an expected outcome. People didn't go around saying their own names out loud on a daily basis after all.

So Roommie, as I had taken to calling her in my head, was all the moniker I had to go by.

Roommie bent over to tie her shoes and I ducked back under the covers and pretended I had never left. I was going to be late most likely. Slowly so as to not disturb the fluffy mountain of duvet I had buried myself under, I slipped my hand under my pillow and pulled out my phone. 8:35 a.m. beamed in my face, only too happy to remind me that I was going to have to rush again.

It was just my luck that my roommate had to have a class at the same time, but it was stupidity on my part that I had been unable to negotiate a solution to my tardiness. A normal person would have worked out timings for the bathroom. I alas did not fall under that category of normalcy. I had chosen instead to pretend I didn't have a class at all and feign sleep while Roommie was around, and then scramble to get ready for a 9 a.m. class as soon as she was gone. Not a suitable arrangement by any means, but I did love my privacy a little too dearly to part with it. The mere idea of dressing myself and preparing myself for a day in front of a campus full of people in front of someone else was beyond even considering.

And whose fault is that?

The soft click followed by a beep let me know that the door had shut behind my intrusion and that I was finally alone. The covers flew off and a dead sprint got me to the attached bathroom so fast I would have given the world record holder a run for his money.

Heh, get it? 'Run'

The rush to clean up, utilize the facilities, dress, and get out the door left me breathless and I was unhappily reminded of the poor state of fitness my body was in, and the monumentality of the pending sprint to campus. Not that I sprinted, the thought of the passing stares such a scene would cause a great hindrance to the consideration of the idea, but it certainly meant I was one of the late ones who arrived after class was called into session.

The indignity of my own incompetence tasted foul as I rushed in when the professor's back was turned. Silently I crept to the back of the class, doing my best to melt into the air as I maneuvered myself to an empty desk panting for breath, a thief in the act of pretending she had not just robbed time. My undue efforts at stealth did not seem to matter; I had either already cemented my reputation as perpetually tardy or nobody really paid me any mind since I made no noise despite the fashion of my arrival and I never showed any intention to participate anyway.

I settled in, pulled my black hoodie up, drew out my notebook and a pen, and set about turning my attention to the lecture. The professor cast a reproachful glance in my direction, the only indication that my presence was acknowledged in the class.

For a class that met thrice a week, the professor was not expecting the stars from the sky when he had asked the class to show up on time. To him, my persistent lateness was an insult to his instruction, clear and simple, and I cringed in shame as his gaze landed on me.

Ha...

He was a tall man, my professor. Neat and tidy, his brown hair touched by sunlight, not a thread was out of place in his appearance. In comparison to his sophisticated presence, I must look like a loach in my black attire, hair disheveled from the hood and not a speck of make-up on my face.

Professor Thomas was a dignified American man in his late forties I'll guess, and he taught with a passion for history and simplified it in ways that blew my understanding of the world out of the water. And he had been infinitely patient with me for the past month.

Hafsa...

Today's history class seemed to be focused on talking about the formation of river valley civilizations, a natural progression after we spent the month discussing the discovery of agriculture and the domestication of animals.

Like I am certain it was for Professor Thomas, history was one of my joys in life, era non-relevant. It was a calculated decision for why I had chosen the course and why the subject had enjoyed reigning championship as my favorite since I was very young. Besides the selfish understanding that as a historian, my career would rarely depend on prolonged or regular human contact, history offered a realm of escape. There was a purity about history.

Hafsa.

History did not require decisions. It did not require constant debate. The actions of our forebearers were already taken, words already spoken. All we had to do was understand what they meant. Understand how to avoid the same mistakes going forward. There wasn't anything else you had to do. No one to talk to. No names to ask. That suited me just fine...

"Hafsa!"

The loud voice drew me out of my reverie and I was unpleasantly deposited unceremoniously back in a hard chair at the back of a dreary cream-colored classroom. The classroom where everyone was staring at me pointedly and I became keenly aware that I had just been snapped into a living nightmare with such force that it chased the breath out of my lungs, like a rubber band being drawn back into shape after being absurdly stretched.

Eyes. There were too many eyes. All of them focused on me, glowing out of hollow skulls, weeping disdain. The classroom dimmed and elongated, as if it was being stretched. The voice that called my name rang through the heavy silence like the echo of a deep-toned bell.

I gasped, trying to get air back into my deflated chest. The air, however, had stubborn plans to remain uncooperative. It was too thin. No, it was too thick.

Again?

I gasped again, fingers extruding out of the oversized hoodie sleeves, tightening on the wooden edges of the desk. A feeble attempt to gain some solid footing in a world that was bent on being bent out of shape.

"Shall I repeat the question?" the professor asked, exasperation toned in his voice like a leaden threat.

Problem's not the question.

The eyes stared, rolling in their skulls like ping pong balls. Red fat tears ran mockingly down my classmates' faces, a mockery of the fact that my own eyes were welling up. For a brief moment I wondered if I would cry red too.

My knuckles were turning white against the painted veneer of the cheap desk. Limbs shaking from a blind need to run, run, run far away from the students who were starting to stare disappointedly, waiting for the one black sheep to pull herself together and move the lesson along. They were starting to fidget. I heard them, toe-tapping, nail-biting, pencil-scratching, head-swiveling. Someone moved their legs and I heard the rough scrape of denim. Another student scratched idly at his beard, the dry *kishk-kishk* of his fingernails grating in my ears. Someone cleared their throat and it was like a grenade went off. It was loud. Too loud and my fingers burned with the aching agony to clap my hands over my ears and childishly block the sounds of life out.

"Can you name a river valley civilization? You should know this."

I did. I actually knew several. The sooner I made that clear the sooner the eyes would turn back away, disinterested. I opened my mouth to answer and…uttered absolutely nothing. The silence rang, deafening, mocking, like heavy fog in a forest. My tongue fled to the back of my throat, like an animal cowering in the back of its burrow while a predator lurked outside. Something in my throat clenched and the feeling of being suffocated multiplied tenfold. I was choking. My lungs burned with the need for oxygen. Help, someone help!

"If you're not going to pay attention in class…"

This time I truly wasn't listening. Fire consumed me from the inside out. It burned!

Here we go…

My hands jerked, clawing at my chest in a futile attempt to assuage the blossoming flames that were swallowing me, a witch being burned at the stake. I pulled off the hood from my head in a desperate attempt to assuage the feeling of being suffocated.

The notebook and pen went skittering to the floor as my limbs thrashed uncoordinatedly, rejected actors in the gruesome play that was unfolding.

"Hafsa?"

Breathe, idiot!

I choked, a guttural croak escaping my lips as I wrestled with the air for territory. My lungs shriveled as they burned like paper in a barbeque fire, eyes freshly watered, limbs shaking, shaking, hands no longer camouflaged by the large hoodie.

I tried breathing in, choked. Out, choked. The ever present darkness that had been creeping in from the edges of the walls now stole the edges of my peripheral vision, crawling forth leisurely to claim the pariah that had been stolen from it to walk the earth in the guise of a human girl. It was coming. The glowing eyes the only things still visible in the dim expanse of the skewed room.

I didn't realize when I started to cry, but when a fat teardrop fell onto the desk and exploded into a dance of colors I found that I couldn't stop.

Stop! Just stop!
Help.

I wanted to hide. I wanted the glowing eyes gone. Something large moved in front of me and I jerked away from it violently, sliding from my chair, knees hitting the tiled floor on my way down with a muted thump, shaking hands latched onto my sternum willing it to expand, just breathe. Air. It hurt. I needed air!

"Hafsa!" the professor rushed over. I heard the terrible *clack-clack* of his shoes as he ran, the squeal of desks as students stood up or moved out of the way. They were starting to panic as well, I could taste it in the air like sour yoghurt. Not quite as blind as my own predicament, but just as devastating in its own way I bet. Someone leaned in to make sure I was OK. I couldn't tell if it was the professor or a fellow student.

If only I could get to my earphones...but they were far out of reach.

I wanted to run. I wished I could melt into the earth. I desperately willed myself to die.

None of those things happened.

But the professor learned not to ask me any more questions.

Chapter Eleven
Silence

Piper was an ass.

I should explain. Piper is a cat I'm fostering. Long story.

Basically, I've always wanted a cat. So much so that I gave in to my parents' insistence to get braces because they promised me a cat afterwards. They lied. But now I have nice teeth. Yay for integrity and honesty.

So when I was able to get my own reasonable apartment in Sharjah, I decided enough was enough. I was getting a cat.

And so I adopted a month old abandoned kitten. Renn. Why the double N, you ask? For pizzaz. No other reason.

Renn is the little joy of my life. A warm hyper little ball of fluffy energy who brings reason to my existence. The little floof even managed to melt my brother's stoic heart. He secretly loves her more than I do but is too macho to admit it.

Renn's everything I'm not: energetic, playful, social, and fearless. In fact, Renn only has one little minor teensy issue. She's a biter.

So when an acquaintance asked for help to foster a 'gentle sweet cat' named Piper for a month, my brother and I actually considered it. It might give Renn some company and teach her how not to play rough. That, and you know I have a hard time saying 'no.' So Piper was dropped off and we quickly learned that we had been sorely misinformed. Piper was an ass.

She was loud, and whiny, and clingy, and a bully. She ate Renn's food, drank Renn's water, stole Renn's toys, and attacked Renn every chance she got.

"That cat has no honor," my brother declared and promptly decided he wanted nothing to do with Piper.

Renn on the other hand, was terrified. So on an early Friday morning as I watched the two cats square off for the umpteenth time, I couldn't help but admire my little Renn. She was visibly shaking, her whiskers and ears flattened back, her little tail puffed to twice its size. But she advanced toward the hissing Piper one slow, hesitant foot at a time. She wanted a friend and by God she was going to make one, even if it was Piper.

Watching my little girl bravely stand up to a cat five times her size and several times her age, I couldn't help but feel connected to her. In a beautiful display of narcissism, I was reminded of myself.

Renn was acting out something I did every day on a mental level. Or at least that's what every day felt like. I would dress boldly, do my face, and strut out of my house as fast as I can so nobody notices that I'm actually shaking or that every step I take, every moment is one test of the conviction of my will after another. When you struggle with Social Anxiety, every day, every interaction is a nightmare to be faced. And like Renn, every day feels like an uphill battle.

Dr. Sameer once said something to me that resonated with me. "You don't have Social Anxiety," he said. "You *live* with Social Anxiety."

And as much as I am loathe to give myself any credit, that part is true. I could shut myself in at home, live with my parents, refuse to go out and face much easier struggles. But I don't. I have a job. I maintain a social life. I put on my performances to get by. I *live*.

Perhaps that is why I find so little faith in therapy. Because no one seems to acknowledge this. The advice I am given most often, by my friends, my parents, my doctors, is that I need to face my fear and get out of the house and do things. Bitch, please. I face my fear every day. I go to work, that's a fear faced. I order food and smile at the delivery boy, that's a fear faced. I meet my friends, that's a fear faced. I go out in public, that's a fear faced. OK so I can't go shopping, that's a fear not faced but hey pick your battles, all right?

I'm not saying I'm brave, believe me. I am perpetually terrified. But at least I try. If I could attribute one word to myself, it would be courageous. Because facing your fear even when you are afraid takes courage. And if that's the life I am going to lead, hey I can think of way worse words to associate myself with. The thing that lets my war slip under the radar is perhaps the fact that I fight my battles in silence. I don't declare that I'm scared, or that I don't want to do this. Neither do I openly celebrate the little victories. I ordered coffee for myself by myself. I saw a movie alone. I went to the mall. I went to work. I didn't feel the need to cut. I answered a question in a meeting, shakily but answered nonetheless.

In a moment of hypomania, or normalcy for me, I once booked a trip to London. I was happy and the world was my large box of french fries to be eaten and savored. I was excited! Until the happiness wore off and I was back in the depths of depression again. The upcoming trip felt like a nightmare. What if I had a panic attack in public? What if I couldn't go into a restaurant to order food? What if I went all the way to London and missed out on everything because I was too scared to actually do anything? I wasn't scared of going alone. I was terrified of going as me.

The trip finally rolled around and I boarded the plane and off I went. Not for the millionth time the thought of cancelling the whole thing crossed my mind. But not only were cancellation charges a bitch, I refused to let the solo trip of a lifetime pass me by. So off I went. And I made sure to enjoy every minute that I could. Did I struggle? Yes. Goodness knows how many meals I skipped because I couldn't work up the courage to go in a restaurant and order fish and chips like a bawse. But I explored in my own quiet little way. Little nooks and alleys and the open moors and the highlands. Hidden waterfalls and soft conversations with other travelers and tour group companions. I took a photo of someone for them and had them take mine in return.

If all of that isn't 'going out of the house and facing your fear' then I don't know what is. Do I need to do improv? Stand up comedy? Act in a play? Go skydiving? Actually hold that thought on that last one. I actually want to do that.

I'm not a saint. There are still things that I don't have the courage to face. I have wanted to take singing lessons ever since I was a little girl. I was too shy to ask my parents to sign me up for them. I even took to singing in my room with the hopes that they would pick up on my interest and ask me if I wanted to take lessons 'cause goodness knows I was horrible. But I never worked up the courage to actually ask for it. And it remains one of the biggest regrets and missed opportunities of my life. I could do it now, but I don't have the courage to climb that peak and actually do it. The thought scares me, and I'm worried about what any instructor would say to a fully grown adult showing up at their door asking for a lesson usually reserved for children in Sharjah. But maybe one day. I am not giving up hope on that just yet.

I've imagined life in the shoes of the people who stand back and let life pass them by because "so and so thing gives me anxiety." I guess I must have always been a fighter because I refuse to let that be me. I can admit when things make me anxious, but I solemnly vow never to allow something to "give me anxiety" ever again.

Chapter Twelve
Acceptance

It was late by the time I was done with the check up and ultrasound and I was leaden with the profound disappointment of learning that my thyroid problem was autoimmune-related and that I was going to have to live with taking daily pills for the rest of my life. Even my body was slowly quitting on me. I felt like a building you watch from your window at night. The lights turning off one by one until the whole structure is a silent, dark shell. Twenty-four was not the age to be feeling that melancholic about your body and mind slowly dying on you.

A loud sharp beep stunned me out of my reverie. A taxi stood parked in front of me, the driver peering curiously out of the passenger window, wordlessly asking if I needed a ride. I did. But I was still perplexed as to when I had actually left the hospital building.

The door tugged open with a rusty squawk and I gingerly lowered myself into the back seat. I softly told the driver the address and settled in to aimlessly stare out the window. Brightly lit buildings whooshed by in a blur of warm whites, fleeting and brief. They danced through the pane of the window like ghosts, ephemeral and hollow and transcendent. Nothing felt real. Not my fading mind or my failing body or these massive concrete phantoms. So when the reverie was shattered into a dozen sparkling pieces blinking out of existence, I was mad at being forced from my state of non-existence.

I blinked, looking for the sound that had disturbed me. It turned out to be the driver talking. Asking me some mundane question about where I was from. Ignoring him seemed to be the right option to choose, and I was not in any semblance of a mood to indulge a chatty taxi driver. Not tonight.

"Where are you from?" he asked, more insistent still, body craning back to look me straight in the eye, one hand roguishly clutching the steering wheel, the other resting haphazardly on the passenger seat headrest. The car swerved dangerously, someone behind us honked, and I feared I would spend my last moments plastered to the road unless the driver turned back around and took control of the vehicle. But the driver seemed resolute to not do any such thing until he had the answer he was looking for.

"Tunis," I muttered, layering just enough of an accent on to be convincing but not too abrupt. The lie was easy, and one I was willing to uphold since this driver seemed to be the chatty type. I was glum at being pulled from my saturnine musings by so unorthodox a method and I hoped the random country would discourage any notion of a conversation. It didn't seem to be the case as the man chatted away about how this was a new country that he had never heard of before.

"Are you married?" he spat out along with a mouthful of spittle as he turned once again, leaving the driving to the mercy of the whims.

"Yes," I quickly lied.

The man looked me up and down in a manner most disrespectful.

"I don't see a ring," he observed.

I stared at him. Was there a point here?

"Huh? I don't see a ring, eh," he repeated, more insistently this time.

"I took it off." I turned my head back toward the window, effectively severing the thread of the conversation and bringing death to the fledgling connection before it devolved into a full dialogue.

The sudden chill that wormed its way under my skin was paralyzing. I whipped my head back to see the taxi driver with his face turned forward but his hand firmly gripping my knee. The sight sent me reeling into shock and I felt the familiar tightening of my chest. My breath betrayed me and my lungs decided to revolt. Air seeped out of the car through the cracks of the windows and doors. My vision blurred, head dizzy and suddenly so unbearably heavy. I tried to speak but it was like my tongue was made of lead.

The hand slowly crawled its way up my knee and the insane itch it brought with it drove me to the very brink of insanity. I wanted to chop my leg off then and there. I wanted to smack the hand away, I wanted to cut it off its parent limb and burn it and scatter its ashes in the sea. But I didn't do any of that. Instead I froze and simply stared at the hand working its way up my thigh. Those fingernails, they're huge. It was an odd thing to notice, but now that it had been noticed that was all I could see. The large flat fingernail of the thumb seemed to grow and expand, the white stained with red from *paan*.

"Move your hand," I choked out finally. The three words were a battle to form, and an even greater battle to utter. But they came out so breathless and so low that it made little difference. If anything, they served to do the opposite. The man turned around again, grinning wolfishly.

"I know you lying," he lilted, his voice singsong.

The band around my ribs tightened further and my mind panicked over whether to address the pain or to address the incessant tainting itch. Everything was going several miles a minute but I seemed to be stuck in place. *Not now, not now, not now! Breathe, you stupid idiot!*

The hand massaged my thigh and the need to set myself on fire was maddening. It felt like the hand with the giant fingernails was tracking mud over me, oozing tar, turning everything it touched filthy and sinful.

"Stop!" I breathed, begging, eyes glued to the fingernail, hands gripping the faux leather cover of the seat under me.

"What?" the man sang leaning back further toward me. The car swerved. The hand reached higher. And I jumped away from the man with everything I could muster, head smashing into the window with shuddering force.

CRASH!

I wasn't sure if the taxi hit something or if that was just the sound of my head meeting with the glass, but the man panicked. The hand withdrew and the driver finally turned his attention back to his job. To my surprise and relief the car slowed and pulled itself to the curb.

Gasping for air, I lunged for the door handle and shoved my full weight against the door. It didn't budge. The lock!

The door creaked open and I spilled onto the sidewalk like jello from a tilted cup. The taxi driver yelled something after me but I couldn't make out the words. *RUN*! My mind screamed at me, a wordless, featureless howl of terror and pain and panic. And so I took off at a shaky hobbling jog, trying desperately to get my lungs to work.

I couldn't recognize where I was, my mind far beyond its capacity to understand symbols and words. All I knew was *run*! And so I ran. At some point I remember palm trees. A brief sensation of running on sand. Was I near the beach or the construction site? I didn't know. I caught a flash of orange and white from the side of my vision, horror gripping my shuddering heart at the realization that the taxi was following me.

I remember nothing else from that night but the next thing I was aware of, I was home. I was shaking. I was crying. And I was terrified.

Cut to a year later and Dr. Sameer was going off on a spiel about my state of mind and I wasn't having any of it.

"Imagine if I couldn't write with my right hand," he began with undue enthusiasm. He gripped his pen awkwardly and exaggerated an epileptic shakiness in the limb to really drive his image home. "I could try, but the writing is going to be unreadable," he explained as he wrote his name in a messy script that would be hard to identify in a pile of four-year-old handwriting practice sheets. "So what do I do?" he asked. It was likely intended to be a theoretical question, but I was in the middle of one of my low dips and I felt the burning need to be snarky.

"Learn to write with your left hand," I muttered at him.

He obviously hadn't anticipated my answer when he began his analogy and it fell apart very quickly in my opinion. "Oh. Yes. OK. I suppose I could do that. But that will take time and it will never be as good as the right hand. So now what should I do?"

"Give up."

Dr. Sameer sighed, and do I detect a faint whiff of frustration in there?

"No," he restarted after a few calming breaths that gave me an unholy amount of glee at making him feel just an ounce of my own frustration. "We learn how to support the right hand. If I help the right hand by supporting it and giving it strength, I can write with it, isn't it?" He gripped his right wrist with his left hand and calmed his exaggerated shaking in order to write his name clearly this time. He finished with an expectant grin on his face and looked up to see the scowl on mine. His lesson had obviously fallen on the wrong side of the fence as far as I was concerned.

Dr. Sameer was telling me to learn to accept that I was lacking something that everyone else had and learn to accept the help that was being offered. That was a fine lesson in and of itself. But I heard something very, very different in between the lines.

'You're permanently broken and you should learn to accept the crutch that we can offer you.'

No. Absolutely not. I couldn't find it in me to accept that. I was looking for a cure, not a crutch. Anything less than absolution meant that I would live with myself forever, till the day I die and then beyond. And that was unacceptable. It was such an easy thing to say when you haven't lived as I have. As others like me have. The taxi incident, as I took to calling it, was fresh in my mind still, the humiliation of the panic and the terror of not being able to help myself was a constant recurring nightmare. Any condition that put me in that situation and rendered me helpless and unable to save myself was something I could not and would not accept. It was that very same incident that pushed me to give treatment another try, because never again did I want to be caught in a situation like that. I would never allow it again. Ever.

What I needed was the ability to say 'No' when I needed it, the ability to think clearly in the presence of another human being. So if a crutch is the best that could be offered to me, then sorry but no. I would hold out for better.

Acceptance was not an option. I refused.

"I'm a shy person too," Dr. Sameer claimed. I immediately distrusted it. *No you are not. You don't care what others think about you.* Wasn't that the prerequisite for falling in the category of shy? Simply being nervous of presenting in front of others was not shyness.

And lying to try and build a rapport with me was unforgivable.

What most people, and most therapists it would seem, didn't seem to understand was how much of an impact Social Anxiety has on your life. How much of your life it steals from you. Experiences that could have been enjoyed, friends that could have been made, happiness that could have been. Alternatively, no one truly understands the challenges that could have been overcome, obstacles that could have been avoided, suffering that could have never been inflicted.

And what? We are to simply accept it as part of us? Accept the crutch and live with the anxiety and the constant terror as a part of our daily lives? No. we deserve better than that. We deserve to be free.

I deserve to be free.

No more.

Chapter Thirteen
Sadness

For the millionth time, I checked that my roommate was out and would not be back for a while yet. I fought the urge to send her a text with the stupidly worded message "Hi, you're not going to be back for a while right?" No, sir. That would make it sound like I was planning to engage in some porn while I was alone.

No, my intentions were much more sinister. I intended to wallow in sadness. A sadness so dark I forgot I was sitting in a brightly lit white room. I always thought the dorms looked like a mental institution's ward. And here I was about to do something mental.

I opened the door to my wardrobe and stared at myself in the attached mirror. A tidal wave of sadness swept over me, a wave so deep that it took my breath away. The world shrank, then expanded, distorted and fractured and held together by sheer force of failing will. The universe turned into a giant eye that stared holes into the fabric of my soul through the mirror. No matter how I try to turn away from it I never can escape its gaze. It sapped the strength from my legs and I felt like I was sinking into the very muck and mire the cosmos was made from. It robbed me of my worth and I knew that in the grand scheme of things I meant nothing. This skinny bitch that stared back over gaunt cheeks and sunken collarbones was worth nothing.

The world had tested me and I was failing in every possible way at every turn. Purposeless, worthless, and unneeded. Shame crept over my skin like slime and I mourned the hour I had been born if all I was a joke to the nature of existence. Guilt for taking up air, food, water, space burned itself into the threads that bound my soul to the earth.

Loneliness burned in my lungs like a fire I had inhaled, and I choked on it. There was no place for me. Nowhere to belong. Nothing to serve. The fire burned hotter, whiter and I ran till the chains around my ankles were winding their way upward. Fear tore at my skin bleeding it dry, a thick crimson sludge that seeped into the velvet black like water after the first rain. So little. I meant so little. What was the point of anything when anything my hands could ever make would be consumed by the blackness of the endless expanse? There was no point. Nothing. Nothingness.

Like me.

Blades were my escape, and blood the baptismal waters from which I would be reborn. The little art knife jerked over the bare flesh of my left shoulder. Like Moses commanding the seas, skin parted. A crevasse, a canyon of white and pink flesh dotted with the seeping pearls of red. The pearls multiplied, intensified, congregated at the bottom of the ravine like lost lambs herded together and it flowed and it flowed and it flowed till the ocean of red wept over my arm dripping to the floor in a steady *drip drip drip*.

The velvet universe shuddered to the dying strains of a piano encore and then the sadness drained away. The feeling left, leaving behind an aftertaste of burned coal and ash and something horribly sour. I swallowed to little effect as the taste lingered on my tongue like residue from an air freshener when you accidentally swallow it from the air. But finally it was quiet. My head rang with the blissfulness of silence, my inner demons shocked at what I had done. I had threatened retribution and I had delivered, a horrible terrible chastising for being the failure that I was. No more empty threats of needles and scratches, punishment would come more severely from now on.

I looked at the girl in the reflection, her eyes bright and glassy as if she had just taken a hit of something powerful and it was doing wonders to her nerves. One arm was turning red as little rivers coursed new paths around the limb, the other hand still holding the art knife blade. Blood tickled as it flowed and suddenly I was floored by the weight of the crushing realization that I had taken a step I could not take back. Crushing sadness and loneliness and self-hatred and weakness and fear, they ran rampant through my numbed mind. What had I done? What had I done? What had I done?! Unbidden the thought popped into my mind. *Well you wanted to die didn't you? Here you go. Now you can slowly bleed out.*

I understood just how badly I wanted to die. And yet, I couldn't completely understand at the same time.

My head swam, high on the endorphins and dopamine and all sorts of other chemicals my brain had just released as an answer to what I had committed against my own body. And I was drunk on too much of it. My ears rang and the little voice I had silenced by cutting came back full force screaming in panic. *You're going to die! What have you done?!*

My knees went weak and I leaned heavily against the cupboard door to stay mostly upright. Not like this; they couldn't find me like this. I didn't even register which 'they' I was worried about.

I reached for a wad of paper towels and pressed them to the wound. Pain lashed out, both pleasant and agonizing at once. I tried to apply pressure but realized my hands were shaking too hard. The steady hands from a second ago were now leaves in a gale. Right hand clamped to the oozing wound, I grabbed for more paper towels to wipe the blood off the floor.

The paper towels got soaked and for a second I worried I had hit an artery or something. A foolish thought considering there wasn't anything on the top of your shoulder anyway. But the fear lingered as my fingers felt the crimson moisture soaking through the tissue. I grabbed another couple and tried again.

It seemed like an eternity before the blood stopped coming and I was ready to pass out. A little bit longer, the little voice in my head cried. Just hold a little longer. How odd, the voice in my head was being nice. Maybe I was already dead. Putting the soaked paper towels in a discarded pile, my blood-stained fingers rummaged in the drawer for a bandage. I always kept them stocked for emergencies such as this.

My shoulder was in agony now. I made the biggest mistake I could at that moment, I turned to look at the wound one last time before I bandaged it. The wound looked awful and angry and accusatory. My vision tunneled and all I could see was the cut. A bout of vertigo gripped me tight and swiped the tiled floor from under my feet. I wasn't even aware I was on my knees until the faux marble pattern was practically wiping my nose. I wanted to vomit, I felt so sick to my stomach. There was an odd aching in my bones that I couldn't explain. My head throbbed, a jungle tempo of boom, boom, boom.

Just a little longer.

I slapped the bandage on, braving a look in the mirror once more to see what I was doing. The girl in the mirror looked like she was on the verge of keeling over. She didn't look pleased or happy anymore. Terror read on her face, plain and simple. Tear tracks stained her cheeks, tears I wasn't even aware I was crying.

Putting my shirt back on was a hassle. I was terrified the wound would start bleeding again with the movement. It did, red staining the sterile pad of the large-sized band-aid. But in the end I managed, and the gaping screaming wound was hidden under checkered fabric. Like magic, the pain receded to a dull throb. My bed beckoned and I was ready to lie down and never wake up again. But the pile of blood-soaked paper towels on the desk needed attention. Cautiously and on fawn legs, I took the handful of bloody refuse and chucked it in the big bin in the dorm hallway outside my shared room. From some deep reserve, I mustered the strength to wash my bloody hands before making my way finally to the bed. I had passed out before my head even hit the pillow.

That was the first time that I upgraded from tiny scratch cuts to deep cuts. I was nineteen and alone in college, far from home. It was a messy affair and the memory of the relief it first brought as well as the ensuing terror left a lasting impression on me.

Now when I cut, I have rules.

Rule number one, never use your left hand.

Rule number two, don't cut again until the last time you cut has fully healed.

Rule number three, no words.

Needless to say, I've broken all my own rules. But I broke rule number three last.

I didn't want to carve words simply because words change meaning over time. If one day I decided I was feeling pathetic and decided to cement that reminder into my skin, it might last for a few weeks or a couple months before another feeling overtakes it. Then I might decide I am a loser. And I decide that it needed to be carved in as well. A few months later I might feel like incompetent is the word that best describes me. And so on and so forth.

The trouble with feelings is that feelings are fleeting. Sure they may last for a while and while they last they may feel overpowering, but it is a lesson in self-control to remember that they are in fact temporary.

A second reason for the third rule was that a scar can be explained away. Oh, I fell off a bike and landed on a sharp rock. Or I got scratched by the cat. But how does one explain away a word? Oh, I was chopping vegetables you see, and the knife slipped and carved the word 'stupid,' isn't that fascinating?

But the biggest reason was that I didn't want those words to win. I could very easily carve in 'stupid' or 'idiot' or 'dumbass,' but I believe in the power of words. Giving such words permanence gives them the reins and I for one am not willing to let go of the reins just yet. I don't want those words to have power over me. And I'm not ready to let them win.

But sadness is a powerful force to withstand and I have not withstood it well over the years.

When I finally carved words, I wanted them to mean something special. Something that would be relevant regardless of my mental state.

When I finally carved words, I was done living and was praying to die.

Memento Mori.

Remember you must die.

Memento mori is a term that I first learned in the history of western art. It is a term that represents the inevitability of death. It's a practice of remembering death that goes back to the Greeks. In art, it's the dying leaves, and the symbol of the skull, and rotting fruit.

But that's not the term I chose.

You see, I remember I must die. What I must remember is that I cannot. If my self-harm is already slating me for divine punishment, then I don't need to add more reasons to sign up for eternal damnation. I was suicidal. But I was not allowed to suicide.

So I chose my words carefully. Something to remind me to keep going when the urges hit and the world dims and the universe tips and light in my soul dies a little more.

Remember you must live.

Memento Vivere.

Chapter Fourteen
Anger

Now, I should be clear; I like to think that I'm generally not an angry person. Angsty moody teen years aside, and usual sibling rivalry battles with my brother notwithstanding, it takes a lot to get my blood boiling. Like my pain tolerance, my anger threshold is fairly high. You would have to call my mother stupid or something equally offensive to warrant a punch in the face. Call me stupid and I'm likely to agree with you.

It might have something to do with the fact that I direct any anger toward myself rather than point it at the world. But that's a finite game to play and eventually your cup is going to overflow.

In my case, my cup finally exploded.

When I was a child, my mother read me a story from the Quran. One of the prophets had the gift to speak with animals. And in this story, the prophet was marching through a valley with his army when he heard the sound of faint screaming. "Run!" it said. "Quickly! Before we are all crushed to death!"

The prophet halted his army immediately and when he looked down he saw hordes of ants scurrying away as fast as they could. The prophet thanked God for giving him this gift, for without it he never would have been able to hear the cries of the little ants.

Ever since I heard that story, I have a habit where I stare at the ground when I walk. I guess that's the little hope that I gave myself; perhaps one day when I'm standing before the Divine in judgment, He would extend his mercy to me the way

I tried to extend it to his tiny creation. I've tried hard to live without accidentally crushing any ants when I walk.

At least, that's the reason I give myself for why I walk with my head down. And in my defense, I don't actually know how much of it is not true.

So when I snapped, it was funny that the thing that made me snap is the one habit I have followed so diligently.

In my defense, the ant was stupid.

It was a sweltering afternoon that found me wandering thoughtlessly back to the dorms after classes were through for the day. It had been one of those rough days that entailed a presentation of my design work to a panel of judges whose job it was to vehemently judge the shit out of my work. Now normally a student can defend their work. I, on the other hand, froze up and let the panel berate my performance and my efforts. The long walk back to the dorms was abuzz with the stir of a hornet's nest of self-deprecatory thoughts. OK so maybe the walk wasn't so thoughtless. Listless more like, as I repeated every phrase I had heard that afternoon over and over and over in my head till I wondered despondently why I was suffering through this major in the first place. I vividly remembered the look my professor was giving me to explain my thought process and explain what I had been thinking when I had picked the concept of a Japanese style pod hotel and designed the hotel restaurant with a ceiling covered with Japanese lanterns. And I remembered his look of disappointment when all I did was stare helplessly at him back, jaw firmly locked.

God, why did I have to freeze? Why at that moment? Why couldn't I just be like everyone else?

It simply wasn't fair. This was the fifth time in a row I had screwed up because I couldn't defend myself.

How could God make me that way? What was the point?

At that moment I paused to let an ant pass, but at the second I put my foot back down the ant darted under my shoe. Horrified, I lifted my foot back up to see the damage I had caused. The ant lay there, twitching in agony and what I at least hoped was regret.

Something in me snapped and before I knew it I was yelling at the stupid bug. Quietly of course, I'm not a madwoman...and in Sindhi.

"Idiot! Did you really want to die that badly? Fine! Die! Did you enjoy it? Who told you to walk under the shoe? I was trying to save you, you moron!"

What I was really saying was something very different. "How could I be expected to live this way? I try to get things done and do what is expected of me, but it wasn't fair that the world insists on fucking everything up. This stupid ant could have lived! I could have passed my presentation! I could be passing my classes! Why did the ant have to dart back under the shoe? Why did only I freeze up during a presentation? Why was my professor such a hardass? With all odds stacked up against me, what was I supposed to do? It wasn't fair. It wasn't fair!"

But in perfect angsty fashion, my day wasn't even over yet. Not by a long shot. I reached the dorms and opened my email to see that I had received a notification about my grades from the last semester. The cumulative GPA was up. And to my absolute horror it had dropped even further thanks to a rotten design grade from last semester, the semester with the professor who liked to hear praises about herself. The professor I couldn't bring myself to suck up to. The professor who just about failed me for it.

I had dropped too low to receive the chancellor's award scholarship. And by a margin of 0.02 points I had missed the gold medal that I had been gunning for three years.

It was over.

If I had snapped at the ant, I erupted like a human version of Vesuvius at this news.

The world was an absolute shithole and I couldn't understand why I was being punished. I was trying my best, but my best didn't seem good enough. Didn't God say he helps those who help themselves? Didn't he say that if you begin, He completes? Where was He then? I was dying trying to do my best and He had yet to show His so-called Grace and His so-called Mercy.

I was trying to do the right thing, I was trying to get by on pure effort alone. Why did I have to be made in such a way that every effort was washed away by the incompetence of my ability to express myself? Why was I born this way? Why was I made to live this way? Where was mercy here when I begged and I begged for God to just kill me because I couldn't take it anymore and I was so exhausted of trying? If He couldn't kill me, could He at least not make things worse?

But my prayers fell on deaf ears. All my begging and crying did nothing. Nothing changed. And for the first time in my life I truly hated God. I hated him for how he had made me. Hated that He was absent and silent. Hated that He didn't seem to care. Hated that my pain meant nothing to Him. And by extension, hated this world He had created and everything in it.

I spent every waking moment seething. I felt like a kettle bubbling with pent up heat, way past the boiling point. I couldn't even tell who I was really mad at. All I knew was that I was in pain and I didn't have a way to make it stop, much less understand why I was hurting. So I lashed out.

Someone cut in front of me in line because I was too timid to say no? They were going to get kicked in the shin "by accident." Someone told me I couldn't sleep in the library? Well then have fun arranging these books that I took off the shelf and left on the table like an ungrateful brat. Someone wanted my notes to cheat off of? Here have them, enjoy deciphering the Sindhi I wrote them in.

I was the very epitome of pettiness. I like to think I was a passive aggressive demon but the truth is petty was all I could manage. And that served to piss me off too. I couldn't even be angry properly because that would involve calling attention to myself. I felt like a horrible caricature of a joke gone wrong. 'Cause that's all I could be, right? A joke to the rest of creation?

Nothing else made sense. Up until this point, I had had faith to rely on. God would help. God would come through. He would not abandon me. God cares when I hurt.

But my faith was dead. Not just dead, it was burning before my eyes and I felt lost without it. I still believed in God, I just despised his callousness. To hell with all the talk of mercy and strength and growth and patience. It was all rubbish. If any of it were true, I would have learned how not to be me years ago. Instead I was progressively getting worse.

And in true helpless fashion, like an animal caught in a trap, I turned all my fury upon myself. God was a no-show, but I wasn't any better. I had failed myself at every turn.

Eventually the rage burned itself out and I was left staggering with an armload of bitter ash and apathy that left me numb. And in many ways that was worse. At least with the anger, I had an indication that I still cared what became of me in the end. With numbness and apathy, there was nothing to gauge my level of emotion.

I had given up, plain and simple.

Part Two: Peripeteia

Chapter Fifteen
The Myth of Exposure, Exposure, Exposure

The reason I started writing this collection of randomly assorted memoirs was so people could get a glimpse at how the socially anxious brain thinks and processes the world. Perhaps you suffer from the disorder and you want to know what other goodies are in store for you down the road. Or maybe you know someone who has the disorder. Or maybe you're trying to explain to your doctor or therapist that this is what is going through your head but don't have the self-confidence or words to do so. In any case, this collection would be incomplete if I didn't offer any of the lessons I have learned over the years for how to combat the condition or offer some insight for what worked and what didn't work.

In my case, therapy didn't work out. Despite all the praise and ringing endorsements for Cognitive Behavioral Therapy, in my case it backfired. I was left feeling more lost, more broken, more irredeemable. Rather than slowly grow in my confidence and assuredness in my own ability to overcome what I considered to be my greatest weakness, I became that much more aware of the gap between myself and the rest of the world. I felt stuck in place while the rest of the world moved on with such effortless ease even if not grace.

So why didn't therapy work for me?

As much as it pains me to say this, I believe it was because the therapists working with me were unaware of how to work with a real live case of social anxiety disorder. They all believed in the power of "exposure, exposure, exposure" but did not know how to administer it in a way that would be received well by people like me.

If exposure was simply the key to solving the problem, we would all be cured by the simple fact that we expose ourselves to the world every day in various ways. Sure we might be about as social as a houseplant, but none of us are hermits living a solitary existence in the mountains with the wolves. We are part of the world, even if we feel apart from it.

That is not to say that exposure does not work. Unfortunately, it is the highway that we must all traverse in our journey out of S.A.D.land. But exposure is only constructive when we are equipped with the right tools. Because our lack of exposure is not the root of the problem. The way our mind is wired is what makes us tick wrong.

Just as you cannot send a soldier into battle without his weapons, you cannot send a socially anxious patient into the world to "go forth and be cured of your isolation."

So let me give you some ammunition that I have collected through my experiences. And I'll see you on the other side.

Chapter Sixteen
First Steps – Calm the Inner Voice

Like most of you, my head is a cacophony of screaming voices. Some are screaming for attention, others with the need for attention, and others still berating me for seeking attention, and still others that simply scream in terror at the prospect of spending yet another day facing the world. Among those voices is Ravenniel.

Remember Ravenniel? My alter ego? Well, at first I thought it was this voice that simultaneously tried to keep me safe from the world by enabling my isolatory and self-destructive habits, and yet screamed forth abuse when I think I have failed in some way. But I have long since learned that Ravenniel is not the only dominant voice in my head and that there is one more alter in there. The one that spews forth verbal abuse with a language that would make a sailor blush. But it was not always this clear cut. In the beginning, there was just me and my usual shame for being the way I am. Just one inner voice.

Dr. Hendricksen calls this inner voice the Inner Critic. And this Critic exists as a misguided way to keep you safe from the social embarrassment and risk of isolation that we fear. It eggs us on to give up and give in and let the anxiety win.

Ah if only mine were ever so thoughtful as to protect me from potential social humiliation. After the level of self-loathing and shame and guilt we live with, it is hard to view this voice as anything but malicious. The bottom line is, I cannot learn to accept this voice as a potentially possibly maybe benevolent-but-misguided attempt at caregiving.

So how to fight this imaginary bully? Why by giving it form, of course, and then kicking its sorry ass. Us Quiet types lead rich inner lives. So why not use that to help us fight?

This is where I tell you what is Ravenniel and why everybody needs their own Ravenniel and how to do exactly that.

You see, the Inner Critic is a formless entity. So what we are going to do is give it form. A form that isn't you. In your head, picture whatever makes you feel lousy. Your third grade teacher. That bus driver who yells at everyone. That kid who bullied you in school. That goody two-shoes classmate. Barney. Heck, a jello blob with three eyes and tentacles. Why not? This is going to be your 'monster.' The ugly side of the Inner Critic.

The next time you call yourself dumb or stupid or a waste of space, visualize it coming out of this creature's mouth. Because next, I'm going to share my embarrassing technique to shut that mouth.

You have your 'Monster,' now let's create the 'Hero.' Only this time, the rules are opposite. I want you to imagine yourself. Picture yourself without your perceived 'flaw.' Imagine yourself as the person you would be without your social anxiety. Or your depression, or whatever you believe is holding you back.

What you just pictured is going to be your Ravenniel. Your very own alter-ego. And this alter-ego is going to be your avatar, your champion in this fight.

I found this exercise helpful in practicing mindfulness. Because ultimately, this is an exercise in identifying negative thoughts from positive ones. "You're a failure" comes from the Monster living in your head.

Now the hard part is practicing self-compassion to go along with the mindfulness and to combat the negative thoughts. And that is where your Ravenniel comes in. Self-compassion is her department. Her (or his – sorry fellas) job is to give you a break, cut you some slack. Battle your Monster and shut it up for a while.

Just as your Monster is powered by your fear and shame and self-loathing, you must be the power source for your Ravenniel. Our fear, despite how we feel, is irrational. We know this. So let your Ravenniel be your rational mind. Challenge the Monster. "I'm stupid? Why? Because I panicked during a presentation? So it wasn't my best day. What of it? How bad was that really? Am I going to die? No. So shut up."

Dr. Hendricksen calls this strategy Replace and Embrace your Inner Critic. Her lesson was that we must learn to Replace the negativity of the Inner Voice with rational thought and question the stance taken by the Critic. Secondly, we must learn to Embrace that the Inner Critic is a part of you and is only trying to keep you 'safe' in the only way it knows how.

But the problem is that I don't want to embrace this voice. In my head the abusive voice and the caring one cannot be reconciled into one entity. I don't want them to be the same thing because that makes it harder to challenge it. I can understand the misguided attempt at keeping me from social risk, but I cannot understand the verbal abuse. Like an abusive relationship, there is too much history there to forgive. So I advocate splitting the positive from the negative, and challenging the negative using the rational and compassionate Positive in the over-the-top extravagant style that is my personal brand of 'creativity.'

If it helps you to visualize an epic Avengers style battle in your head where your heroic Ravenniel single-handedly takes on the big bad Monster, go for it. Whatever floats your boat, bro. Or if you prefer a battle in a courtroom. Or perhaps a wild west showdown. Sure, you might feel silly as a grown-ass adult imagining a battle in your head but guess what? It's only in your head. No one else can see. And as far as my paranoia has taught me, mind readers don't exist.

Now you may be wondering; how exactly does this help?

Well, for one, it taught me that I am not at the sole mercy of my thoughts. I can learn to channel them and challenge them, even if I can't control them just yet.

It taught me that mindfulness can be more than meditation and yoga and breathing exercises. I'm far too imaginative for meditation to really work, but an epic anime-style battle between the forces of good and evil for the freedom of my soul? That I can do.

In time, I started noticing myself emulating Ravenniel. If you haven't guessed it yet, the Ravenniel that you imagined for yourself is the true blue authentic you. And that's the idea: to free 'you' from underneath the chains of whatever you believe is holding you back.

In time, I also started noticing that I was kinder to myself. The idea of self-compassion seeped through the cracks of the Monster's walls and armor.

But this only works if you keep one thing in mind: you have to try. Ravenniel is not magic. She's powered by you, remember? (If you imagined your Ravenniel as a superhero then oops. You can keep that image, but the concept of Ravenniel as an alter ego is still not magical) You need to put the conscious effort in, no matter how silly it feels at first. And in time, like any good character arc, your Ravenniel will start to grow stronger.

And so will you.

Chapter Seventeen
Become the Hero of Your Own Story

So you've now managed to challenge your Monster. What next? Now that you have successfully confined your inner demons into a personified 'Monster,' and the helpful side of the Inner Critic into your alter-ego, your Ravenniel, it's time to take the next step.

There was a reason I asked you to picture your Ravenniel as yourself. Because she is you. She is what you want to be. And she is what you can be. She is the power you have within you. And now that she has the ability to be more in control, she is what will guide you forward. So in a really simple method, you are going to become your Ravenniel.

The next time you are in a situation that makes you antsy or nervous and makes your skin crawl, ask yourself "what would Ravenniel do?"

Your Ravenniel. Not mine. Just checking yeah?

Ravenniel is you without your anxiety, remember. So what you are really asking is "what is it I wish I could do right now?"

In the beginning, I started out doing that for small seemingly simple things. Standing in line at the grocery store. Waiting in queue at the coffee shop. Standing in the elevator with another person.

To be perfectly honest, at first the exercise made me quite miserable. Ravenniel would stand with her head up and look at the check-out clerk in the eye. Ravenniel would not be afraid to stand off to the side and take her time to make a decision first before joining the queue. Ravenniel would cross her ankles and lean against the elevator wall because she's tired from the long walk.

But why couldn't I do any of those things? All that exercise seemed to prove to me was that I was incapable of doing even those simple things.

But if you push through that hopelessness and pain, the exercise does have a point. It helped me clarify and visualize what I wanted to be. And how I could do that. Pixel by pixel it helped me build a clear picture of myself without my debilitating anxiety that I have had all my life. The problem with having the disorder since a young age is that we think in the wishy washy wish of "I wish I didn't have social anxiety." But how well do we know what that means really? What is life without social anxiety? What does it look like? If we cannot remember a time without it, can we really imagine that life clearly?

I would argue, no. If we are really honest with ourselves, we don't really know what not having anxiety feels like. We simply want it gone. But a clear picture is a clear goal. And that's what the suggested exercise did for me. It helped me build a better picture of what I really wanted.

And in time, when I was miserable enough, I noticed myself beginning to ask a different style of question. *Why* couldn't I do any of the things I wanted to do? Rather than why *couldn't* I do any of the things I wanted to do? It's a subtle difference, but it's there all the same.

And with this little change, I decided to try to act like Ravenniel. I held my chin up in the grocery line. I looked the clerk in the eye as I put three bottles of diet Pepsi on the counter and dared him to lift an eyebrow in judgment. I stepped out of line and stared up at the menu board, taking my time to decide what I wanted to get before rejoining the queue. I leaned my frame against the elevator wall tiredly, even if I didn't have the badassery to cross my ankles just yet.

Ultimately what I did is the same principle as power-posing. Only, you're doing it with your mind. Research has shown the effectiveness of power-posing for a few seconds in order to improve your confidence. Now imagine how effective it would be to do it with your mind.

When I went for the presentation skills training course, I was told that the course was designed to stretch us out beyond our comfort zone so that when we go back to our daily lives, the shape we settle into is bigger than the state we started out in. The only problem was that the process of stretching was fast and sudden and painful and I don't deal well with being pushed into the deep end. It's the same with therapy. It calls for exposure and practice and like it or not, it is exposure and practice that's ultimately going to make a difference. The problem is that exposure and practice is often dumped on us by our therapists. Dr. Marie tried that and Dr. Sameer tried that. This method is slower, gentler if I may, but ultimately does the same thing.

In time, the simple exercise of emulating my Ravenniel in little ways began to feel more comfortable. So slowly, I moved on to bigger challenges. Ordering food at a restaurant. Disagreeing with a close friend. I began by asking what I wanted to be able to do, and when I had a clear picture, I tried to follow that picture. And then when I could do those, move on to even bigger challenges: making a point in a meeting, going to a movie alone, answering the phone. Rinse and repeat.

But over time, it began to work. Things that seemed hard in the beginning became easier over time and repetition. So why did this method work when previous attempts didn't?

The answer is where it begins to get a little boggling so stay with me here.

You see, people like me are uncomfortable being ourselves. I'd argue that that was the case with me because of my sense of guilt for being broken. And if it is rooted in the sense of self-loathing and failure then it might be a feeling shared by others with Social Anxiety. So why not be something other than ourselves? A better version of ourselves. Just different enough to help us slip into character but at its core, still us.

The ultimate fake it till you make it cheat card.

Chapter Eighteen
The Difference Between Roles and Personas

At this point you're probably thinking, and rightly so, that wait a minute…isn't faking it till you make it a lying strategy I use? And didn't it *not* work out for me? How hypocritical of me to suggest it again.

How is what I'm suggesting different from the characters I play?

And you would be right to be confused, for the line between what I do and what I am trying to suggest is very fine at best. The difference here is a question of roles and personas.

In her book, Dr. Hendricksen talks about roles and fake fronts. She points out that people suffering from Social Anxiety often face difficulty in forming human connections and maintaining social interactions because, more often than not, there is no structure to guide the interaction. To combat this confusion, she suggests giving yourself a role. By giving yourself a role to play, you are creating the structure to guide us. This role could be as an advocate for a certain cause, a sister, a mother, a friend.

But there is a difference between a role you assign yourself and a persona. A role is a support structure. It comes from within you. A persona is an act designed to fool or distract. If a role is a support structure, a persona is a facade.

And that is what I do. I use personas, put up a fake front. I lie.

When I first raised the issue of my personas to my doctors, both Dr. Brian and Dr. Sameer did not see what the problem with them was. To them, I was 'getting out there and faking it till I made it' like a seasoned pro. They did not seem to grasp the sense of guilt and inadequacy I carried because of it and the fear of the fact that what people saw in me was a lie.

Yes, in a sense I am 'faking it till I make it,' but the problem lies not in the *faking* part, but in the *it* I was faking.

Think of it this way. I am looking for a job and I have a bunch of interviews lined up. Obviously I want to make a good impression. So in order to do that I dress in my finest. Each interview I go to I perfect my outfit and fly fashion sense until I look like I could be designing outfits for magazine covers. My first impression is flawless. But oddly, I'm not getting the job. Why? Because I've put all my attention into what I look like that I have neglected to perfect my resume, my portfolio, or what I say in the interview. I am not faking the needed confidence or experience. Oh don't judge me; as if you have never floofed yourself up in an interview before.

And that's the major problem with a persona. Unlike a role, my personas don't come from me. My personas are based off of characters from popular media. Or based off of people I know. In terms of cultivating an authentic sense of self or growing comfortable in my own skin, I'm doing zilch. Absolutely nothing. All I'm cultivating is my ability to put on an act.

This in turn leads to the exhaustion, the increased pressure to be perfect, and the heavy guilt of living a lie. So to the therapists out there, do take personas seriously. Because not only are they exacerbating the problem, the dependence on them hinders any progress.

And to others out there like me, don't make the same mistakes I did. The sad reality is that personas and acts work. Very few people we meet and interact with everyday seem worthy of our delicate and fragile selves. So who cares if I act like Daphne from Scooby-Doo or the Terminator? But the truth is, at the end of the day, none of the people you interact with will have to live with you (unless you have a husband or a best friend or a roommate or something I guess). But you do have to live with yourself.

So assign yourself a role if you think it will help you. Today I'm going to be the person who asks the barista for whipped cream on my coffee. And do it. As you, not as Daphne.

And if you can't be you yet, that's fine. Be the better you. Be your Ravenniel.

Chapter Nineteen
What to Tackle First

You know how when you put earphones in your pocket? And then they're just a ball of tangled mess when you pull them out again? Oh don't give me that; even if we're moving into the era of wireless earbuds now, you started off with the wired ones. Bite me.

It's nothing less than a form of magic I tell you; if you have figured out the secret to untangled earphone wires, do a public service and share that shit.

Now add another pair of figurative earphones to the metaphorical pocket. Do your fingers curl at the mere thought of trying to untangle that?

But what if you add a third? A fourth?

Now for the part you so did not see coming. Your struggles are the tangled ball of earphones. Original right?

Being the complex human being that you are, it is not only quite possible, but quite probable that you have more than one thing going on with you in your life. I know I have a laundry list of things that I suspect are wrong with me. But you gotta listen to the music of life right? That's why we all walk around with earphones. Otherwise you gotta deal with people.

Just let me have my analogy. Not so bad now is it?

But when you have a hopeless mess of wires where you can't tell where one pair of earphones stop and another pair begins, how do you start to unravel the ball of often volatile issues? Where do you begin? I doubt even the more experienced therapist always nails this the first time. Sometimes you begin unraveling one wire only to hit a dead-end. Or worst case scenario, make the tangle worse.

Now I am not a therapist, but I don't jump on the bandwagon of 'we will work to unravel everything slowly.' For one, that answer is vague as hell. And second, I am not convinced it is doable for a single therapist to tackle multiple problems all at once. And in some cases, perhaps not advisable. Let me give you an example.

When I started therapy with Dr. Marie or Dr. Sameer, they both tried to handle the self-harming behavior and the social anxiety all at once. What resulted was me trying to overprocess the trapped emotions since self-harm was cut off along with the anxiety of exposure therapy. It became too much and I ended up suffering from a rather volatile phase of major depression lows and even reverted back to suicidal thoughts. Not only is tackling too much hard to manage from a therapeutic perspective, but can you imagine how overwhelming it is for a patient? Behaviors and habits are set in concrete if not in stone, and trying to manipulate them is a potentially dizzying psychedelic whirlwind of change at an elemental level. There is no harm in taking things slow.

I know a big wrench in that plan could be something as fundamental and mundane as finances. Goodness knows I struggle with the prospect of "ah, another session next week eh? Sure; I'm made of money." I really hated it every time my doctor told me that "we will get to that so and so issue in the future." I've been in regular therapy for a good year by the time I write this and I can promise you we haven't touched on 5% of everything we said we would in this future that never comes.

The thought certainly frustrates me. I mean I'm paying good money for help but it feels like that help is always something over the next hill. And then over the next. And then the next.

You could argue that there is a dark side to psychiatric therapy and the evil influence of capitalism cheats you out of getting the help you need. And there is certainly merit to that claim.

I will also bet my right foot that "yes we will get to that…later" is a therapist's go-to answer when they don't know what to do yet and are trying to stall for time.

Perhaps a more forgiving way to look at tackling issues in therapy and the ever-persistent 'later' is that therapists are only human. Which basically means that they forget that they promised to tackle a particular issue. And to be fair, can you blame them? They see multiple clients, all with weighty issues like yours. And then there is the time between sessions. If you have weekly sessions, it is quite a bit to ask a therapist to be able to remember a promise a couple weeks later. I mean I barely remember what I did this morning, much less something I said a week ago. I know people who would argue that if they are paying a therapist, then they are expecting the therapist to have a viable long-term plan. And that's certainly not too much to ask. It is part of a therapist's job after all to develop a treatment plan. And I say therapist's job because in cases such as mine, it is not realistic to expect the client to always remind the therapist of a promise they made. In my case, and perhaps in the case of other Social Anxiety patients, my illness keeps me from reminding my therapist of an issue we promised to tackle. Simply put, I am afraid of the therapist's judgment for bringing up the issue again. What if he thinks I'm being impatient? What if he thinks I'm focusing on the wrong issue? What if he thinks I'm telling him how to do his job and he doesn't appreciate it? If you aren't bogged down by fear of judgment and *what if*s, feel free to talk to your therapist about an issue you would like to address. Remind them. But people like me can't do that, regardless of whether we trust our therapist or not. As a therapist, it falls on you to keep track of your promises and follow through on them. So therapists, I'm looking at you for this one. You gotta step up your game.

But assume you have the magical therapist who does actually have a long-term plan but you still never seem to get to the point where you 'tackle the problem.' Could you then perhaps be more open to the fact that perhaps you are just not ready to tackle that issue yet according to your therapist? I know I was not. I was certainly frustrated at the time, but in hindsight I discovered it would have probably done more harm to tackle an issue I wasn't ready for.

Which brings me full circle to my original point: take things slow. Tackle an issue at a time. Will that be any easier? No. Will it cost you a pretty penny? Yes. But does it have the most potential to help you in the long run? I would like to think so.

So fine. Take it one issue at a time. Now you may be thinking "but Dumbass, I got 99 problems and the one we are tackling ain't one."

First off, thank you for that. Second, that's a very realistic concern. And it happens a lot. Like I said, I've been seeing a doctor steadily for over a year now, and I feel like we are not tackling the right problem at all. Will I one day have the courage to say that to my doctor? God knows. Miracles happen right?

But if we are agreed that perhaps tackling one issue at a time is a safe and correct approach, the question remains of which of the earphones wire in the tangled mess we should unravel first. I think I have an answer for that. Now this might differ from person to person and case to case. But I would argue that the first thing you should tackle is the depression, if you are suffering from it.

It's a sad statistic that Social Anxiety Disorder and depression often go hand in hand. And if you think about it, it does sort of make sense. If you suffer from Social Anxiety, you are more likely to be self-isolated. You are more likely to cut yourself off from the world and the activities that strike terror in your heart. Connections with other people are hard. So we grow lonely and trapped in our own heads. And that is a perfect recipe for depression. There is probably a statistic somewhere that this percent of people with Social Anxiety also develop depression over time. But I am too lazy to track down that number and this ain't that sort of book. Soz.

Now there is a reason I picked depression as the earphone to tackle first. Well, several reasons actually.

To start with, depression is very much a hindrance that impairs daily living. Depression has a tendency to make simple tasks that much harder. The effort involved in getting the simplest things done, to focus, to pay attention, to do anything really is absurd when you are depressed. So riddle me this: how are you expected to put forth the courage and effort it takes to tackle your Social Anxiety if you are having trouble finding the strength to put your sock on? Just an example. Maybe you don't wear socks. I don't know.

Second, in the case of social anxiety, or at least in my case of social anxiety, depression served as a source of confusion and distress. There are days where I can't get out of bed and I am unsure whether it is because of the anxiety of seeing other people or whether I simply can't find the strength to get up. And this has the tendency to do something worse: enable. In the case of the previous example of trying to get up in the morning, the depressed mood and corresponding lack of energy served as an excuse to not try and get up at all. Goodness knows how much trouble I have gotten in at my job because of this. And I know for a fact that if I wasn't spending so much energy trying to muster up the…well…energy and resolve to do simple tasks, I would have more to devote to fighting my Social Anxiety. You only have a finite amount of fucks to give, and if depression starts sucking them all up like it tends to do, then there is less to give a fuck about the things you are responsible for.

Related to the confusion and distress, the sort of numb apathy that depression brings to your doorstep makes it really hard to actually *try*. Why would I bother putting in the effort to do my therapy homework when I really can't be bothered about anything. Apathy shuts you down, which means you are not really actively receiving anything that the therapist is trying to give. Think of this apathetic state as a doorway. Depression and the numb apathetic state that it can bring with it is the equivalent of shutting the door. If you can't be bothered, you're not likely to try to actively get better and that makes this state a major brick wall in your attempts at improvement.

Fourth point: depression can sometimes become severe enough that it warrants being tackled first. No, it becomes necessary to tackle first. Not only does tackling it first keep it from sapping all your energy and resolve and courage to keep going, but tackling it might be the key to keep you going at all.

In 2018 I hit a rather low point. And I mean *low* point. You know the one I mean. In my case, when I become severely depressed, I start thinking of ways I could 'accidentally' die. I get to suicidal pretty fast, with the only thing holding me back being the thought that it is outright haram in my religion and God knows I don't need another reason to go to hell.

But that 2018 December I got low enough that the mere thought of celebrating the coming of a new year full of more misery and strife and struggle filled me with dread and despair. I couldn't take another year of this. I wanted out.

So I would start engaging in risky behaviors, such as not counting the number of pills I was taking, in the possible hopes that I might overdose and die. Or stepping into the street when the traffic light is not quite on the little green man yet, in the hopes that a driver would be in a rush and be saddled with slow reflexes to boot.

When your depression hits that low point where you are actively seeking out a quick demise, however underhanded or subtle your methods may be, the Social Anxiety sort of takes a backseat. I mean you are literally threatening your very existence and livelihood. At this point the depression has no other option but to become a priority. You can't fix your tangled ball of wires if you set fire to it all.

Finally, out of all the issues Social Anxiety brings to the table, depression is the one that actually can be helped. There are medications available that can help alleviate at least some of the symptoms, allowing you some breathing room to focus on other things, such as the Social Anxiety or self-consciousness or self-esteem or what have you. If the help exists, you might as well reach out and take it. You can think of refusing help when it is available to you like those people who refuse to take cold medication when they have a raging runner. They insist that they will get better on their own. Or they "don't like meds." You know the person I mean. I don't get them either.

Unlike cold medication, there are actually reasons for concern with antidepressants. My parents refused to get me psychiatric medication because they "didn't believe in it" and "the side effects are too severe." And you know what? I do see their point somewhat. To someone who reads the side-effects on the leaflet, the list can seem daunting. And there is valid concern. After all, antidepressants mess with stuff in the brain, an absurdly delicate balance of wiggles and wrinkles and tissues and chemicals. Messing with that balance is something you should definitely consider before taking antidepressants. In my case, I couldn't understand this reluctance to enhance the chemical balance in the brain. I mean it obviously wasn't so balanced after all considering it wasn't working like it was supposed to anyway.

And besides, antidepressant medications have come a long way today. I mean we're not living in the dark ages.

Think of it this way: if you have the faintest glimmer of hope that something can give you a fighting chance in your long and taxing upcoming battle with the Social Anxiety Monster, isn't it worth taking it? Depression is a parasite of a monster in and of itself. If you can pluck that leech off, I'd say do it.

Chapter Twenty
The Roots of the S.A.D. Problem

So we know where to start maybe. That's great. We know where to start untangling our mess. But if you take a moment to think about it, we haven't really solved the problem, have we? Life happens. And the next time you pull your earphones ball out of your pocket, it's going to be in tangles again.

'Cause ultimately we have not been taught how to roll up our earphones so that they won't tangle. Or for that matter, we haven't been taught that perhaps we could untangle our wires and then put them in different pockets. Compartmentalize and structure our mind to handle life in a healthy manner.

I am loving this analogy. It takes itself places.

But my point is that there is no point in untangling the same wire over and over again only to put it all back into the pocket for it to get tangled again.

Let me explain in perhaps another way.

It's not going to come as a surprise to anyone when I admit that I am not great in front of a crowd. That doesn't mean I am a bad presenter, but it does mean that my brain runs on hyperspeed with hyper-awareness of my surroundings and myself. I become acutely aware of the fact that my voice is shaking or that my hands are trembling or I feel like I'm going to fall. And the moment I become aware of myself doing these things, that is all my mind is going to think about. An endless repeat of "my hands are shaking, everyone can see, my hands are shaking everyone can see, my hands are shaking." So in order to get through the torment faster, I speed up and race through my presentation so fast that my words jumble up and

I end up not quite making the point as clearly as I was trying to make.

This is different from not having presentation skills. I have taken enough training courses to be able to recite what makes a good presentation. Build a rapport with your audience, maintain eye contact, use your gestures, body language matters, voice modulation, structure your content. And on and on.

Now you could argue that, Hafsa, there is a difference between knowing something in theory and being able to do it in practice. And you would be absolutely correct.

Except that I have a counterargument to that: I am held back from practicing the skills I know due to the physical symptoms the anxiety causes. So ultimately exposure therapy falls short because the physical symptoms don't necessarily go away over time. The mental strain or anxiety can alleviate, sure, but in my experience the physical symptoms remain.

And that's where exposure therapy falls short. If you get a diagnosis for Social Anxiety, chances are you have been told that you need to expose yourself to social situations in order to gradually reduce your fear and anxiety. The only problem is, you're most likely told to do this without being given any coping skills for the things that make Social Anxiety so distressing to begin with. At least, a good therapist wouldn't send you out blind and empty-handed.

Anyone with a physical tell or tick can attest to how mortifying it can be in public. Your pits sweat, or your palms get clammy, you flush, your hands shake, or whatever your demon. Now turn that up on crazy steroids and you get a sense of how devastating these symptoms can be for the socially anxious. Someone who is already hyper-aware of themselves and their context.

And you have to acknowledge the fact that physical symptoms are the first thing to get noticed. Especially something as conspicuous as a shaky voice or trembling hands. Imagine trying to point at something in a presentation when your finger can't stay still long enough to actually point at the bloody thing you are trying to point at. Oddly specific?

Yeah busted; that has happened to me. Learning to control the physical symptoms, or learning how to manage them effectively so they are not a hindrance or distraction, whether for ourselves or for others, should be a good place to start therapy work.

The physical aspect is simply one aspect of the shortcomings of how Social Anxiety is tackled therapeutically. There are a slew of other problems with the way Social Anxiety Disorder is understood and addressed. And that has to go back to the first few chapters where we tried to define Social Anxiety and what it is.

Pop quiz time. What separates Social Anxiety Disorder from shyness?

I'll give you a minute.

Remember how we talked about the socially anxious person being afraid of being proven right: that there is something wrong with them that will cause others to judge and reject them?

So let me ask you this, and I'm going to go back to my analogy of the tangled mess of earphones in your pocket. Oh hush, that analogy is clear and you know it.

A shy person would be apprehensive about taking their ball of wires out of their pocket for fear of being judged for the mess. A socially anxious person will avoid taking the ball out entirely because they believe there is something inherently wrong with their wires at a fundamental level. I believe that I don't deserve to take my earphones out of my pocket. Because my earphones will not contribute anything of value by being taken out, regardless of whether someone judges my mess or not.

So with that mindset, how far do you think therapy is going to go?

"Hafsa, I want you to go to a grocery store every day and get used to purchasing a small object."

Yeah OK. But why bother? It's not like I deserve the object. So why would I put myself through potential torment and heightened anxiety situations, if I believe there is something wrong with me at a basic human level?

If I believe there is something wrong with me, why would I risk exposing it to the world through exposure therapy? Why would I risk getting judged for something I know is wrong within me?

With Dr. Sameer, his first exercise was to make me practice public speaking. Surprise surprise.

What is it with social anxiety therapists and public speaking anyway? Seriously? It's not like everyone goes around giving structured speeches every day. It's an old method and it doesn't cover the most basic problem of Social Anxiety. Let it go.

And the basic problem is this: I got up and gave the doctor a perfect speech, using all the skills I know and have learned from training courses over the years. But none of the training, or the public speaking with Dr. Sameer addressed the belief that I am incapable of giving a speech. Nothing addressed the belief that I am terrible at calming myself down, or keeping my hands from shaking, or my voice from quivering like an opera singer. And that ultimately these flaws in myself are what make me a terrible presenter. Unless you teach me vocal control or muscle control first to get a handle on the physical symptoms, a beginning-middle-ending structure of a good presentation is going to do jackshit.

Here comes my crescendo: exposure therapy does not address the core belief that 'something is wrong with me and everyone will find out and reject me for it.' It does not address the self-image and the sense of shame for being the way we are. And unless you address that first before tossing us out into the melee and expecting us to find our way around by 'practice' and 'faking it till you make it,' therapy is going to do what it did in my case: fail.

Remember when I passed public speaking with flying colors, and I was upgraded to trying to empathize with and learn from people around me? I was told to observe my surroundings and study how people interacted with each other? Remember how spectacularly that failed?

Knowing what you know now, it might seem like an easy exercise in perfect vision hindsight to see just where the therapy approach went wrong. I was thrown out figuratively into the world without having any groundwork done to ensure I had a solid sense of self. I was told to observe others without being taught to accept that I might be mentally ill but that there is nothing inherently 'wrong' with me. And with nothing to contest my belief, observation supported my mindset that if everyone else can make connections so easily while I can't, despite having the skill set, then there is obviously something wrong with *me*.

So you can understand my reluctance when I read about studies done with socially anxious patients, or about glorifying exposure therapy or Cognitive Behavioral Therapy. The crucial first step of Cognitive Restructuring is sorely missing. Address the thought patterns first, the self-image, the shame, the sense of self-worthlessness. Then teach how to control the physical symptoms.

And then chuck us in the deep end when we have mastered all that.

Chapter Twenty-One
Pick Your Battles

One thing I have noticed with my personal struggle with Social Anxiety is that problems have a way of compounding.

I am scared of interacting with people, so I avoid them. I isolate myself from people, so I get lonely. That makes me anxious and overwhelmed, so I become depressed. I struggle by myself in solitude, so I learn to hate the idea that there are others out there like me. I feel ashamed of my behavior and my thoughts, so my self-worth and self-esteem plummets. This makes me become more scared of people judging me, so I become obsessed with certain aspects of my appearance. That preoccupation drives me to self-destructive behaviors, which in turn further harms my self-image, which worsens my depression. Which aggravates the need to self-isolate, which begins the whole cycle again.

Trying to solve all the problems at once is like pulling at every thread trying to unravel a tapestry. And we have addressed the issue of trying to root out the core issues. But as with all things, you can't fix everything. Or at least you can't fix them all at once.

What I'm trying to say is this: prioritize.

Ultimately that depends on each case.

In my case, every therapist or doctor I saw seemed preoccupied with my self-harm behavior. The cutting seemed to be the most startling revelation to them and they each jumped on the opportunity in the first session to immediately prohibit me from doing it again. In every concurrent session, that seemed to be the first question asked; "have you cut?"

I began to dread that question because answering it made me feel like I was letting my therapist down every time I answered "yes."

And I get it. Self-harm is a behavior that is difficult to understand, not unless you have engaged in the behavior yourself. In theory, you are hurting yourself. How could that possibly be OK? The thought of inflicting pain baffles most sane people. And inflicting pain to feel better? How could that even make sense? Isn't it a contradiction of everything we have grown up believing?

Well, yes. It's not normal behavior. No one claimed that it was. And that is precisely why most people don't know how to deal with it when they encounter it.

I would go so far as to say that most therapists don't completely understand the need or drive to self-harm. They may know it in theory, but it really is one of those things that's one thing in theory and another in practice. They can read about how people do it for the pain, but how far can they truly empathize? At least that has been the case in my experience.

The constant and persistent nagging about whether I had magically stopped doing it yet just because they told me to stop, told me that my multiple therapists did not quite understand how to deal with the issue at all.

I once worked up the courage to ask Dr. Brian why I should stop self-harming after he had asked me about my cutting for the sixth session in a row. To my dismay he laughed and chuckled "Isn't that something you should figure out for yourself?"

Admittedly, not the best response to give a socially anxious person who now feels judged for asking a sincere question and will probably never ask another question again for fear of being laughed at. Thanks, Doc.

I guess my face must have fallen a thousand miles because he immediately backtracked and told me some nonsense about how as a doctor he cares about my well-being.

Needless to say, the answer didn't sit too well with me. It did nothing to convince me. And they weren't the words I needed to hear. What I needed to be told was that as a human being I deserved to get to a place where I didn't feel the need to self-harm to feel better. That as a human being, I deserved to be happy. That I deserved to be free of the *need* to self-harm in the first place.

Granted my shit self-esteem won't let me believe that right away, but that is where I need help, isn't it? Help me see that I deserve to be happy without the scars, that as a human being I deserve to get to a space where I don't need scars to feel beautiful.

Sound familiar?

It should. We are back at square one. Self-Image. Self-esteem. The alleged root of the whole problem.

I guarantee this, solve this issue and people like me will not feel the need to self-harm. That is a massive bold claim isn't it?

Let me elaborate.

I don't want to stop cutting.

But, Hafsa, aren't you trying to get better? What gives?

Yes. But I use cutting as a coping mechanism. And I am not ready to give it up. Not unless I am absolutely convinced that I no longer need that coping mechanism. That it has been replaced by something just as effective if not more effective.

By simply telling me to "exercise self-restraint" and not do it anymore, you are taking away the only way I have to cope with the dissatisfaction I have with my circumstances, without really giving me something else to rely on in exchange.

A favorite question for therapists to ask regarding self-harm is this: did it make you feel better?

And the long and short answer to that question is yes.

The next question honestly feels more like a backtrack than a well-formulated reasoned argument. "Yes, but did it make you feel better in the long-run or did your problems come back?"

Generally I chalk this up as a silly question. It's a little bit of a silly question that assumes that in life your problems don't come back once you address them. Which we all know is simply not true. Life is life. Problems always come back.

Or new problems appear. It's practically the law of the universe. The finiteness of problems is simply not a good way to gauge progress in mental health I would think.

The second reason it's a failed question is because how else do you explain my case where the long-term effects actually ended up being a positive self-image? Each case is different and not all will have similar results, but the punchline is the same. Self-harm is certainly physically harmful, and it's startling at a human level, but it may not be the biggest problem on the plate. As a therapist, or a friend, or a parent, you might just need to let it go until the underlying problems are being addressed.

Third, I have been self-harming for a very long time. It's become as second-nature to me as changing my clothes. As such, it has become something I am no longer ashamed of doing. In the beginning there was certainly guilt at marring my mortal coil. But as time went on and I learned new ways to justify my behavior, the guilt has dissipated. True that I won't go flaunting my scars in public, but that is more from the avoidance of unwanted attention and questions than actual shame. Convincing me that it is a behavior that is objectively, or even subjectively, wrong is going to take months or years of effort on the therapist's part. Couldn't that time be better spent addressing issues that need to be changed and are willing to be changed?

Again, case by case. I know I am lucky enough that I am in control of my self-destructive actions. Remember my rules…that I broke?

For a lot of people out there who are struggling, control is very sketchy at best when it comes to self-harm. They might not be able to help pushing the limits too far. If a person is a danger to themselves, by all means, address the self-harm. But provide ways to cope without it. Cold turkey does not work with medication, it does not work with habits that are so deeply rooted that they have taken hold.

But back to the main issue. So if my answer to the "does it help" question is yes, both long-term and short-term, then as a therapist or a friend or family member you would be buckling down to exhaust a lot of energy in trying to convince me that I need to stop something that I see as a compounded second-tier issue at best. You can get the sense by now that our brains are stubborn forces of nature. If I don't want to stop self-harming, there is very little in actuality that you can do. You will exhaust yourself till you are blue in the face from talking before you begin to make a dent in my mindset. That time could be much better spent teaching me how to love myself, how to grow in confidence, how to build my self-esteem, how to be myself without feeling the need to jump into character.

As these things change, the secondary behaviors should begin to follow, with some help and guidance of course.

Understandably, that is the longer and more difficult path, but in my experience it points toward being the more rewarding one. So for now, pick your battles. I'm asking you to save certain battles for another day. In this individual case, the self-harm. That does not mean you ignore it completely; do touch base on it and check up every once in a while and you should see a pattern emerge as we make progress in our core issues, whatever that may be.

I've chosen the hard path to recovery. I'm asking you to help me overcome the biggest mountains, not to pull the rug out from under my feet when I'm barely standing.

Chapter Twenty-Two
Give Us Hope, Not Crutches

Having talked about choosing a path to recovery, I must now admit to something that is bound to make me very unpopular. I don't believe in a full recovery. I firmly believe 'almost normal' is the best we can manage. Grim? Yeah. But find me something that proves me wrong. Every book I have read, every recovery story I have come across mentions the same thing: the second we are put in a situation that social anxiety doesn't like, all the feelings come roaring back.

Ultimately if I read between the lines, all that means to me is that complete recovery is an illusion. And that by itself is disappointing as hell. Not only am I broken with the hyper-awareness of being broken, I can look forward to no hope of being normal. The most I can be offered is a sort of 'better.'

Now, I would like to believe that not all of us are so naive. We do believe in the recurrence of problems. Like I said, problems don't always go away. I would say people like me are afraid of that. It is actually one of our greatest fears; that we will never get better. That we are doomed to live out our lives as broken. And to me that is more terrifying than say an upcoming presentation or social event. Just the long-term grind of constantly trying to keep your head above water.

And that is what is going to make your job as a therapist, or a friend or family member very difficult. Because I am going to ask you to help me, help us, see the silver lining. Help us find hope. Help us find purpose to keep fighting and keep going. Because otherwise, what is the point? If we are never going to be fully OK, why bother trying so hard in the first place?

I wish I had an answer to share. Something that my experience has taught me that lets me know it's all worth it in the end. But I don't. I'm sorry. I am looking for my point and purpose too. And that is where your loved ones and support system become important. Because I suspect the truth is that there is no cure-all answer to this problem. Every person has to find their own reason for fighting, their own reason to strive to get better. Because no reason or answer I can give you will ever be important enough *for* you unless it comes *from* you.

That was quite nice. Aren't I a genius?

But there is a fine line between finding hope and giving false hope. And this becomes rather important for therapists. What I am asking for is for you therapists to find the humanity in yourselves and be honest with us. If you do not know how to address Social Anxiety as a disorder, let us know. Don't do it wrong like Dr. Marie, or offer a crutch like Dr. Sameer, or drag out and put off therapy like Dr. Brian. I have wasted years in 'therapy' because the doctors were unaware of how to deal with Social Anxiety Disorder but were too stubborn to refer me out or tell me the truth.

"We'll beat this," Dr. Brian's mantra rang at the end of every biweekly session. But how we will beat this, he didn't really know. And as a result I kept going hoping he would one day devise a plan, and he watched helplessly as problems built on problems and I spiraled ever deeper into a problem he couldn't completely understand.

"I used to be just like you," Dr. Brian declared in one of our early sessions. "I used to be very shy."

In all honesty, that should have been my first warning sign. We have discussed the difference between shyness and Social Anxiety at length. Shyness is a personality trait, social anxiety is a distortion. The fact that he did not know the difference should have been my marker to walk away. But I fell prey to the false hope his statement represented; that one day I too could be capable and normal just like him.

As time passed and I failed to respond to his ministrations, I witnessed his confidence change from "I used to be just like you" to "you are a unique person" to "there's a lot of fear and anxiety. I didn't know that before."

And the further my confidence fell.

And the more I wish I had received honesty in the beginning so I would have spent more time searching for a specialized therapist.

If I were to be so bold as to give a piece of advice I have learned, it would be this: find a therapist specialized in Social Anxiety Disorder. Therapy without the specialization tends to spin its wheels in the sand without really moving forward. Especially stay away from the ones who claim "they have an interest in social anxiety." In my experience what this translates to is "I think it would be super rad cool to meet a social anxiety case, never met anyone before." 'Cause I cannot imagine someone meeting one of us and walking away from the experience going "aw swell, that was awesome, dude."

But I get it. Sometimes there just isn't anyone else. And you have to take what you get. In which case, this next part is for the therapist 'interested in social anxiety.'

Move beyond the social skills training boot camp. What social anxiety patients lack is not social skills. Contrary to the popular belief perpetuated by social media and an outdated understanding of the disorder itself, patients suffering from social anxiety are actually very adept at social circumstances. We're no social butterflies, but we observe, handle, and respond to social cues better than anyone else. Remember, social anxiety is a fear of being ousted as 'weird,' so we put our best feet forward in any social interaction. The last thing we want to do is come across as odd, so we make sure we play our parts perfectly. We would not be able to accomplish this without an intimate understanding of social norms and cues.

Like I said, I'm an excellent public speaker in theory. My problem was never the skill set. It was in the execution.

Dr. Sameer's perspective was that if he gave me the skills, the execution would follow by itself. A crutch of sorts.

And I refuse to accept that as the best that is available for me. Just like I deserve to feel beautiful without the scars, I deserve to be comfortable in my own skin in a social interaction rather than molded to fit an external standard of social perfection.

The problem with teaching skills first rather than comfort in self-acceptance is that it enforces a standard for success or perfection that is based on external factors. It takes away a measure of success from our own actions and puts it in the hands of a third party: society. Instead of gauging our growth by our own progress, our success and growth becomes judged by a checklist of dos and donts. And that should not be the measure of success. You should be that measure. Only you. Not an offered crutch.

We deserve better.

Chapter Twenty-Three
Acceptance

"You have to," Dr. Sameer insisted.

My answer was simple. "No."

"You have to accept it," he motioned vigorously with his hands to drive the point home.

"I don't want to."

"You have to accept that Social Anxiety is a part of you," he drove the point home.

"I can't."

My experience with Dr. Sameer is probably quite common. When I started therapy, I thought I had reached a point where I could accept that I needed help.

It wasn't an easy feat. It took time to learn to admit that I was not like everyone else. That I lived with a shackle around my ankle and that my life story would contain a struggle that not very many people knew or could empathize with. Or even understand.

It took even longer to learn to accept that. Let us be honest with ourselves, it is not easy to accept that you are lacking in some way. Especially when the illness itself is the fear that you are lacking in every way.

So when Dr. Sameer insisted that I needed to accept Social Anxiety was a part of me, I was initially confused. Had I not done that? Was the fact that I was sitting in a patient's chair at a clinical psychologist's office proof enough that I had come to terms with my daily condition and that I was willing to fight it to get help? What else did I need to prove?

As it turns out, that is not what the good doctor was aiming for at all. In his professional opinion, I had not fully accepted the reality of the situation.

"It is a part of you," he repeated.

And I finally understood what he was trying to say.

He was trying to make me understand that while I am not my Social Anxiety, it is a part of my unique model and make. It doesn't define me, but it is nevertheless a large part of my life.

And therein lay my problem.

How could I draw the line between my illness and myself?

I had always distinguished my own identity from the social anxiety part of me. It was something distinct, something that had attached itself to me like a leech or a parasite and was haphazardly sucking the living out of my life.

What Dr. Sameer was trying to say went against all of that. He was trying to teach me that this 'parasite' wasn't necessarily something external. That it was just as much a part of me, perhaps so ingrained that it may even be written into the very code of my DNA.

Whether Dr. Sameer was right in his approach or not is not for me to say, but the approach quickly pointed out two very key things that made me so reluctant to buy into his words.

First, his approach took away my drive to fight. By treating my Social Anxiety as something external, I had given myself a reason to fight it. It was after all something that was stealing its way into my life. Stealing my reason for living. Stealing my right and access to happiness and fulfillment. How could I not fight it? But by making the anxiety a part of me, I lost that motivation. It was me after all; what hope is there if you are fighting yourself? If it is a part of me, why fight it at all? Isn't this how I am supposed to be? What chance is there of changing something so fundamental about yourself?

And that brings me to my second point. If Social Anxiety is a part of me, that means it can never go away. If it is a part of you, then how can you ever rip it out or scrub it clean? I began to think of it as a mole, a blemish, or a taint on your face. Hell, why not. Make it a big hairy mole, not one of those beauty marks.

You can surgically remove one of those things, but the mark of it always remains. A permanent reminder that you had this mole. In a sense, you will always have that mole.

What I'm trying to say is this: by making Social Anxiety a part of me, I lost the hope that it is something that can be cured.

I have long since grown out of that notion. I have come to understand that my Social Anxiety is not something that can ever be fully cured. Understand it, but not yet accept it.

And if we get right down to it, how can I accept it? If your journey through life has been saddled with the shackling restraints of Social Anxiety, then you can empathize with the struggle that it has been. You can understand how it has thwarted you at every turn, bested you at every move. A life with Social Anxiety is one of pain and loneliness and self-loathing.

How can we possibly accept and learn to live with something that has brought us so much suffering?

Why should we?

I do not have the answer to that. I don't know why we should accept something that has not only brought us pain in the past, but is promising to continue to bring us misery in the future.

Will it make our lives any easier? I don't know.

But there is no denying that it is a tricky line to walk. Especially as a therapist. Perhaps this is one of those things that needs to be evaluated on a case by case basis. Some people may benefit from accepting their Social Anxiety as part of them. Others like me might fight it.

I have always thought that by fighting the anxiety and refusing to let it have a modicum of space in my life and identity, I was being strong. Perhaps I was wrong. Perhaps that has been the source of my self-loathing all along.

I just don't know.

I doubt many of us know. But as a therapist, I am asking you to help us navigate this part. It might not be the first thing you do. It might not even be the second. But it does need to be something you should address.

If we must accept our Social Anxiety as a part of us, be clear with us. What exactly are we accepting? Are we accepting that we will never be cured? Help us deal with that because I doubt any of us would take that news very well.

It is true that there is no 100 percent cure. Social Anxiety will always rear its ugly head and you will always have moments of weakness regardless of how old you grow and how much therapy you entertain. Any therapist who tells you differently is either lying to you because he wants you to keep coming back or he doesn't really understand his job.

But if you do understand your job, help us navigate this minefield. Help us find peace, whether in acceptance or in taking up arms. But please, please do not let it become a defining part of who we are.

Chapter Twenty-Four
The Problem of Culture

Now this is a chapter that is long overdue and I am going to try my very best not to turn it into a long rant about the nonsense idiosyncrasies of our culture.

I come from southwest Asia. Or as I like to call it, Backwards Land. Nation of the Backwards in Coming Forwards. Land of the Purely Foolish.

I'll stop. I think I have made it abundantly clear that I am rather unpatriotic when it comes to my social heritage.

The reason I am rather unforgiving of my culture is that I believe it had a large part to play in screwing us over.

For as long as I can remember, "what will people say?" has been our household mantra. And by household, I mean everyone extended, removed, and distant. My parents were the worst at this.

My father is probably the most self-conscious person I know. From the way he talks, to how he walks, to how he dresses is all dictated by what others would perceive him. Down to his smile. I personally believe my father has a dazzling smile. One of those honest smiles, you know what I mean?

He apparently doesn't. You see, he has a gap in his front teeth, a tiny barely perceivable gap. But for as long as I have known him, he smiles with his lips together so that people don't see the gap in his teeth. Which honestly makes him look rather awkward. But heavens forbid because "what would people say? Look how the gap-tooth is laughing."

And I wonder where I get my self-consciousness from, eh?

My mother decided to get a little more classy. "I can't wear that color! It's like putting a red bridle on an old mare!"

What would people think?

It was on constant repetition. My father taught my brother and I to always dress our best because we don't want people to think we're slobs. "It's for our self-respect," he stated proudly after he explained why he wears a watch and a pen whenever he leaves the house. "What will people think of me if I dressed poorly?"

My mother expanded the horizons of 'other people's opinions' a little further. "What will people think of your parents if you behave poorly?"

At first I used to think my parents were extremists. But it wasn't long before I realized that this was how they were raised. Their parents put them through the same ringer, and their parents before them and onward.

The truth is that Pakistan is a classic example of an Eastern collectivist culture. Society comes first and then the individual. You are responsible for upholding the image of your family and household name, not just your own. Your actions reflect on your parents' upbringing of you.

What will people say? What will people think?

Do people actually say something? The sad answer is, yes. They do. Very boldly and openly. The problem with handing the reins of your reputation to society to judge is that society will enthusiastically judge the heck out of it. People talk. Everybody talks.

When the Taxi Incident happened, I was given the option to report the driver to the authorities. But the old mantra of what would people say forced me to hold my tongue. Victim blaming and shaming is very much still a part of our culture unfortunately. And once there is a taint on your reputation, it takes nothing short of a miracle to wash it off.

Our culture sucks. It was never intended to foster the self-conscious or the meek. Susan Cain's Quiet Revolution has yet to reach this part of the world.

"People are going to eat you up, dear," my parents often warned me. "You have to be bold and strong."

You have to stand up for yourself, but not too much because people will start to think of you as stubborn or hard headed or hotblooded.

Be firm in your gaze and your stance, but not so strong that it is unwomanly.

Be independent. But within your limits as a woman.

There's no such thing as a mental illness, only weakness on the person's part.

Our culture continues to remain predominantly conservative in a progressively more liberal world.

In many ways, whenever we went 'home,' whatever that is, it never felt like we were living in the twenty-first century.

We are a culture of gossip and back-talk and judgments because we have given society the right to determine our individual value. And society has not treated that responsibility with respect. In short, it is a culture that proves a socially anxious person's greatest nightmare: not only are people watching you but they are judging and their judgment indicates your value.

The most disorienting part about it was that the acute concern for what other people think turns on and off by some subjective mechanism. Sometimes it was life or death what other people thought. Other times no one could be the least bit bothered. And no matter how much I tried, I could never decipher the code for when it was which scenario, to care or to not care.

As much as I wish I could advocate a complete break from such a social culture, I am aware that that is simply not a feasible solution. I wish it was. I was lucky in that I grew up away from this culture and only had access to it through my family and a one-month annual visit. Heh, you could say that itself was enough, heh. But in all seriousness, I cannot even begin to imagine the torment of the socially anxious in such a cultural atmosphere. Or maybe everyone is just secretly socially anxious but they do a much better job of hiding it than I can manage. Wouldn't that be something?

How to address this though? That is the killer question. I don't know.

For therapists, don't bother wasting your time trying to convince us that no one is judging or that the judgment doesn't matter. We all know that is not true and you are going to have an uphill battle on your hands trying to prove anything otherwise. Instead teach us to handle scrutiny well. And equally importantly, how to handle the occasional inevitable rejection. In a healthy manner. Obviously.

For friends and family? Chill with the judgment. *Log kya kahenge* (what will people say) is so last millennium. Instead teach us how to be our own person and to stand up for that person.

Teach us to let people talk if they really must.

Chapter Twenty-Five
Nobody Is Looking

I can be a real asshole sometimes.

The first time Dr. Marie tried to convince me that nobody thought I was worth a second glance, I decided to make life a tad more difficult for her.

"Ah, I see. I am so worthless that I am not worth anyone's time at all. Makes sense. So if I am not worth even a passing glance, why am I bothering to do anything at all? Would anyone even care if I died?"

She balked at that and I gave myself a high five under the table. I think you can appreciate by this point that I was not a fan of hers after her rough treatment during the elevator incident. She can have a field day backtracking till the end of time. I get that it was poor wording on Dr. Marie's part. But it was still an overly rough approach for someone whose self-esteem is a dried eggshell and who operates with self-consciousness on steroids. And like I said, not a fan.

The truth of the matter is, I only half meant my comment as a jest. Because of my Social Anxiety, my self-esteem is already in the gutter. Trying to further convince me that I am not worthy of someone's passing glance simply reinforces the notion and serves to kill off any remaining self-respect I have left. Seriously, If I am not even worth a cursory glance, am I worth anything at all?

Does anyone else have this problem? No? Just me? OK.

The second problem with this approach is that you will have a hard time convincing anyone of this as a legitimate fact. Because it is simply not true. We live in a time where people-watching is a socially acceptable pastime, and as we have discussed, we live in a culture that thrives on watching. So you expect me to believe that nobody is looking? Fat chance.

Big brother is always watching, right?

No, the biggest issue with this approach is that it is misdirected.

Most of us are wildly aware of the irrationality of our fear and feeling that someone is watching us and judging us. We know that in a day we do not really leave lasting impressions. In fact we make sure of it.

We know that the grocery store clerk has hundreds of people passing through his till every day. He doesn't have time to remember you, much less judge your purchased selection. If he did raise an eyebrow, he certainly isn't going to remember it. Embrace a moment of sonder; that guy has his own life and problems to dedicate more than a passing glance at your selection of ice cream and diet soda. Oddly specific example? Yeah, sue me. Cramps. Nuff said.

For the most part, we are quite aware of how irrational our fears are. We just can't seem to stop.

The point of the exercise shouldn't be trying to convince us that nobody is looking. You can't make that promise. And all it takes is one time when someone looked for your entire credibility as a therapist to take a nosedive in my book.

The point of any exercise should be "why does that matter?"

Quite a lot of this is going to have to battle the realities of our culture. How do you argue that being observed does not matter and that people's judgment does not matter when our social standing and social future is dependent on what others observe in us? From the job interviewer who judges us based on appearance and presentation to the eagle-eyed aunties who hunt for prospective daughters-in-law at public events and functions, being watched and being judged is a huge part of what doors are made open to us.

No, the training should not compromise our commitment to putting our best foot forward. Instead it should teach us when to put our best foot forward. When you are uh…in the market (I'm sorry) for a spouse, then yes. The judgment you will receive at a public function or gathering based on how you dress, how you act, what you say does matter. Put your best three feet forward, by all means.

I wish I could tell you that your value is determined by you and not by anyone else, but that is simply not true where we are from. That's not our kind of culture and like it or not, we are born into it.

But on the other hand, going to the grocery store? The judgment does not matter.

But you could argue that if you make a bad impression on the clerk then he is going to make things awkward for you every time you need to check out. Valid. But there is a counter to that. First off, you would have to be an A-grade asshole for a clerk to go out of his way to make life difficult for you. Second, a clerk's priorities are in your pocket. They want your money not your goodwill and friendship.

What I am trying to say is that socially anxious people have their impress-o-meter turned on to max at all times. And that is a stressful and exhausting way to live. Every passing glance and judgment must be favorable and perfect. The person who glanced at us on the street must think I have it together just as much as our inner circle of friends or our spouse.

And that is where we need help. Help us to distinguish where we need to turn our charm on and where it is not necessary.

So I locked eyes with a stranger in a coffee shop. So what? So the person in the elevator I shared spent an unholy amount of time staring at my outfit. So what? So the office boy looked sideways at me when I walked by. So what?

These situations don't matter. Help us to see that. Help us to learn how to turn off the self-consciousness when it is not needed. By learning how to turn it off when it is not needed, we can save our energy to devote it to other far more important things.

Dr. Hendricksen proposes that we learn to ask ourselves the question "How bad would that be?" when we feel like we are about to go on a fritz. It is a solid strategy. But it does take practice. By rationalizing with ourselves and being open to the honest evaluation of the effect situations can have on us, we can learn to let go of our tight-assed self-critical self-consciousness for the moments that don't really matter in the long run.

And maybe, just maybe, in time, we can even learn to digest rejection. 'Cause let's face it, not every evaluation of us is going to be favorable. That's life. Can't please everyone.

But pleasing everyone should not be the point anyway. As long as we are pleased with being ourselves, it should be worth it.

Right?

People are looking. That's what people do.

Teach us to process that and ask "So what if they are?"

Chapter Twenty-Six
Body

With a very simple phrase, what began as a simple movie night among cousins devolved into a horrific timestamp of proof that humanity really is a piece of shit.

The middle-aged actress in her comeback role after her pregnancy appeared on the screen and immediately was greeted with a cry of "Oh my God, she has gotten so fat!" and "Wow, it looks like the TV screen is about to burst!"

No one seemed to remember the fact that she had just given birth. As far as everyone in the room was concerned, she had broken the norm of what she was supposed to look like.

The ridicule was brutal. And with each utterance of "The ground shakes when she walks!" I sank further into my seat.

If this was how people treated someone they didn't even know, I was paralyzed by the thought of how they talked about my chubby ass behind my back. It was no secret that for my physique I was a little on the heavy side. And it was even less of a secret that I got teased for it by my cousins and friends.

If a famous actress was not immune to such ridicule, what would people be saying about my multiple belly rolls?

The thought became fixated in my head. I couldn't get away from mirrors. I absolutely hated the reflection I saw, but I couldn't stop scrutinizing. My belly was the main object of my dissatisfaction.

I was fixated on how it stuck out like a fat little duckling. Or how it rolled when I sat down and stuck out like a bicycle tire. It was so obvious, everyone could notice. How could they not?

My body was a blemish, an imperfection. I was already a failure and an imperfect person, and now I was stuck in a body that reflected the hideousness of my inner world. If I was self-conscious before, it was nothing compared to this new obsession.

I retaliated by cutting down my meals to half their portion sizes. And when I moved to university, I cut those down to absolutely nothing.

I had never had a very healthy relationship with food. I always felt that I was too much of a failure to deserve the luxury or sustenance of food. As soon my physical body got involved, it upped the ante on that thought. Food became a way to punish myself for my failings, both physical and social anxiety-related.

Over time, I stopped eating entirely. And whatever I ate, I took to vomiting back up. There were days I would not eat because I didn't feel like I had earned that right. And then there were days where the social anxiety would keep me from making a phone call to get food or go to the store to get food.

I started losing weight rather drastically as a result. Nobody seemed to take notice that it was abnormal and everyone was so easily convinced that it was just because university life was tough. In my mind, that translated to approval. I got compliments on my physique for the first time and the notion made me ecstatically happy. Lose more. I must lose more!

What brought that to a screeching halt was finding out that with my behavior could classify as an eating disorder if I lost too much weight. I was almost 5 foot 6 inches, and I weighed 54 kilograms. I was in the underweight category and getting close to being severely underweight even though I did not think I looked it. I looked normal as far as I was concerned. But the thought of having something as scary as an eating disorder looming over my head along with my lifelong struggle with social anxiety? That was not going to fly.

So I started eating again. Just a little at a time. And throwing up when I felt I didn't deserve the food or if I overate. I maintained the weight with extreme prejudice. And for a long time that was enough. I never really learned to love my body the way it was, even when I started cutting, but at least I was on some level of balance.

Unfortunately, as things tend to do, it all fell apart. Surprisingly when I started seeking help for my depression and anxiety. The culprit was the antidepressants.

For months I had watched the weight creep on in a kind of fitful denial. Until my weight finally crossed from the underweight to normal category. And all my bad eating habits came rushing back with such force it shook me to my core to imagine how I had been living in university.

So I did the mature thing: I told Dr. Brian. He nodded sagely as I told him about my struggle with food and that I was ruining my teeth with the constant throwing up and that my voice was changed because of it. Finally he decided to change my medicine to a "weight-neutral" one as he claimed, and suggested I see a nutritionist because "this could be a problem down the road."

Down the road?

Down the road?!!

Hello, excuse me. No. This was a major problem now. Not down the road. Not later. In fact the problem was already deeply rooted and engrained since decades, with the abnormal eating behavior about eight years old and running. There was no down the road. We were there already. I had just taken too long to ask for help.

But asking for help and the subsequent lackadaisical response did force me to think about what could have caused the renewed misplaced interest in how I looked. I have always separated the struggles of my physical body and my mind. They were such separate things, how could they be connected? Or so I thought. I certainly know better now. For me, my lack of self-esteem, poor self-image, and rampant self-consciousness were a ripe recipe for my mental issues to leak into the physical world.

As far as I could understand, my body-image issues were linked to my Social Anxiety self-consciousness. If people were constantly watching and judging, the first thing anyone would focus on would be the physical appearance. My drive for creating the 'perfect' illusion extended to the way I looked, and the fact that my antidepressants had taken that control away from me was tormenting me.

"Don't link them; your eating and the social anxiety. Don't link the two," my friend suggested when I confided in her. And perhaps there is wisdom in her counsel. But for me the lack of medical answer was slowly eating away at my sanity.

It seemed like no one was as freaked out by my behavior as I was. Dr. Brian's response that it was an issue certainly, but nothing more wore away at my mind. Without a medical reason for why I was doing what I was doing, I was simply a crazy person.

We're living in the twenty-first century. O.S.F.E.D. is a thing, even if I don't qualify for any of the other eating disorders. But disordered eating is and should be cause for further concern regardless of whether your patient fits into the major categories of eating disorders or not.

Take it seriously. For God's sake, don't treat it as a future problem in development. If your socially anxious patient is bringing the issue up then it is cause for concern. Now.

And take the time to dig into the issue further. For better or for worse, it might be connected to the Social Anxiety. In which case it might affect how you approach the issues.

This should apply to any other problem that crops up. For me it was my relationship with my physical body. For others it could be something else. The point is, if it is brought to your table, take it seriously, please. Don't leave us to think we are simply losing our minds. Hell if the label helps to keep our sanity, then be willing to give it.

Anything but leaving us in our heads alone.

Chapter Twenty-Seven
The Butterfly in the Cocoon

Have you ever watched a butterfly trying to emerge from a cocoon? Or watched a chick hatch out of its shell?

Yeah I haven't either.

But I do have a point to make.

When I was a kid, I read in my school textbook that watching a chick trying to hatch out of a shell is almost painful. The chick struggles and struggles. And any empathetic watcher will want to give a helping hand and pluck the chick out of its cage. But by doing so, you have doomed the chick. Because by struggling through its hatching, it develops and builds the muscles it needs to survive later on. If we intercept that process, the chick never fully develops and will die young.

The same went for butterflies. If they don't use their wings to break out of the cocoon, their wings never develop the strength they need.

Now I am not sure if science has disproved that yet, but the lesson certainly left quite an impression on me.

You are not going to like this chapter, but this one is for all the people out there like me.

Unfortunately for all of us, this same lesson about the butterfly in the cocoon applies.

We may hate our lives, but sadly nothing short of us getting out of our corner is going to fix anything.

My first day in college studying design, my professor tried to instill an important lesson in his class of young impressionable minds. Design, he said, can be an unpredictable thing. Sometimes you control it, sometimes it controls you. Sometimes it goes in a direction you were neither expecting nor aiming for. When you begin a design, you have to allow the process to guide you. You don't start with an end destination in mind. That can be very uncomfortable. How can you make something when you don't yet know what you're making? That's the art of design. You have to learn to navigate that discomfort in order to guide that process. You must learn to become comfortable being uncomfortable.

Granted my professor wasn't quite so eloquent, if I do say so myself. But his lesson rings true for more things than just design. I daresay, his lesson can be applied to us trying to beat Social Anxiety.

Anxiety has a way of forcing us into a corner. A way of convincing us that the miserable little corner we barricaded ourselves into is comfortable. And that leaving that corner will be terribly, excruciatingly uncomfortable.

The self-isolation we inflict upon ourselves as a way of keeping ourselves safe is familiar. We should note that there is a subtle difference between familiar and comfortable. You could argue that there is comfort in familiarity, and you certainly would not be wrong. But neither would you be fully right. The familiar is comforting, but I wouldn't say it is comfortable. I mean, think to yourself; are you happy? Content? Satisfied with how your life has turned out? Chances are if you are reading this, the answer to that question is: No.

Think of familiarity as a baby blanket, or your favorite shirt when you were young. It might be comforting to have it now, but it won't really be comfortable anymore would it. We need to learn to grow into our own size to find true comfort. And that is going to take effort and more than several ventures into the uncomfortable.

The point I am trying to get at is that if you are sick of your life with Social Anxiety, you *are* going to have to make a few changes, a few excursions into some pretty serious discomfort.

That is your phase of trying to bust out of your cocoon. You can have friends who can help you, but no one can do it for you. And unless you do it for yourself, nothing is going to change.

Remember the friend I meet for the Tim's Sessions? Well, for the whole year we met regularly, I would always urge her to order for me when we got to the counter. I was there with her, but I rarely opened my mouth. Until the day finally came when *I* had to go order for the both of us instead of my friend. And I realized that despite having seen my friend do this a hundred times, I was no more able to do something as simple as place an order for coffee than I was when we came here the first time.

I hadn't tried by myself. I used my friend's presence as a crutch, and therefore had not given myself that chance to grow. I used my friend as a comfort rather than allow myself to learn to be comfortable. And the day of reckoning came. The day of reckoning always comes.

I understand it's hard. Believe me, I understand. But I also know it is worth it in the end.

Take it step by small step. You set your own limits and you follow them. As long as you are moving forward.

Can I get up to do an impromptu speech in front of a crowd on the fly? No, of course not. I am not there yet. (Is anyone ever really there? Like really?)

But at this moment in time, can I order my own coffee? Two out of three times, yes. Was it easy? No. Not at all. It was uncomfortable getting there. I made blunders. I made a fool of myself multiple times. I often got the wrong order or said the wrong order or ordered something that wasn't even on the menu. All horrible nightmares. But I got there in the end. I can now order a frozen french vanilla for myself, by myself.

And that feeling of stretching your hard-earned wings after a struggle? Definitely worth it. Go forth my pretty butterflies.

Chapter Twenty-Eight
Panic

This is an interesting chapter to write. Mostly because I have very little input to offer other than what has worked for me. Now that I have set the bar appropriately low, let's dive right in.

Panic attacks.

I won't go into detail about what they are because chances are, unless you are a baby boomer generation or you have been living under a rock, you already know what they are. It's your fight or flight reflex tripping over itself and face-planting in the dirt with its ass in the air. Yeah I am not sympathetic to my under-evolved brain not being able to figure out a threat from something that is not a threat. The brain has had several million years to evolve and learn; it has no excuse.

I honestly can't remember the first time I had a panic attack. But I do remember growing up and thinking I was either just stupid or I was dying from a horrible illness that I was too ashamed to talk of. If I think back to it, that black-out when I gave that speech in the debate competition in Pakistan was probably one of my first few panic attacks.

Naturally as I grew older, they got progressively worse. My voice shakes, my hands vibrate, my head spins, my knees collapse, everything gets hyper-aware unbearably loud, and a vise tightens around my lungs and I stop being able to breathe. Not feeling like I can't breathe or I can't get enough air; I mean a 'no air in, no air out, choking on your own spit, drowning in pain' kind of unpretty.

Glorious times.

So it doesn't come as a surprise that being the enterprising little overachiever that I am, I searched desperately for something that would help me get my own body under control.

What helped me was music. Anything with a steady loud percussive beat that you can time breathing to. I have a whole playlist on my phone titled 'Loud' for this very purpose.

If I feel a panic attack coming, I make it a point to try to get away if I can, plug my earphones in, and play my music from the Loud Playlist on the loudest volume possible. Now I don't recommend the high volume, mostly because I would really rather not be deaf by the time I hit thirty. But this was the only way I ever found of drowning out how loud the world gets when I have a panic attack. The whisk of fabric, the whoosh of breathing, the wetness of words, the dry *kishk* of skin. It gets too much and I need to disconnect from it to focus on getting my body back to a normal rhythm. Drowning the world out in music and breathing to the melody seemed the best way to go about it.

If that works for you, you are welcome to have it. I hope it gives you some modicum of control.

I have been told meditation is another way to control panic attacks, but to be honest with you, it hasn't really worked for me. I can't get my brain to shut up long enough to focus on whatever meditation makes you focus on instead. It takes practice, but it is one of those things that helps in the long run, not so much in the immediate moment.

In time I learned to suppress panic attacks for long enough that I could get away to a bathroom or someplace by myself before it unleashes. To be perfectly clear with you, I don't know how I do it. I just imagine my anxiousness as a pressure cooker that I slap the lid on top of. It doesn't always work. Sometimes my voice will shake and that throws me off, or my hands tremble and that makes me more antsy. But I can stave off the rocking-crying-in-a-corner wreck for a while at least.

When therapists start talking about exposure therapy, I bet for a good lot of us, one of the first thoughts to cross our mind is this: what happens if I put myself out there in some social situation and I have a panic attack and make a total fool of myself?

You wouldn't be alone.

The most terrifying thing for me about panic attacks, besides the whole feeling like you're dying thing, is how unpredictable they are. They come out of nowhere with very little warning. Sometimes it happens, sometimes it doesn't. There's no logic to them, or purpose.

And that's precisely why therapists should make it a priority to help mitigate their effect or the terror they bring if a patient says they suffer from panic attacks.

Because if you don't, I have no safety net against one of the most powerful fears of an anxiety disorder. If there is a threat of possible panic attack in public, you can be sure I am not going to follow your advice and venture out into the socialsphere for the needed exposure or whatever.

My own therapist kept promising to start me with deep muscle relaxation therapy which he claimed is supposed to help. But it was one of those empty promises that never came to fruition. In the end, I was too afraid to step out in public to follow his therapy because I was too terrified of suffering a panic attack. Therapy became a waste of time all around.

Please don't let that happen. Give us something against these disruptive and scary demons. Teach us how to beat it, how to handle it, how to overcome it. How to endure it.

Teach us how to reclaim our bodies from it. Teach us how to reclaim the lives they have stolen away from us and left us fearful.

Chapter Twenty-Nine
Imprisonment

I swear I'm almost done. Hang in there.

This is the last thing I am going to ask all of you sane people out there to do.

Please, get us out of our heads.

Not to be an angsty teen again, but Social Anxiety has a tendency to make you feel imprisoned in your own mind. Unlike the unanxious introvert who can turn their socialness on and off for occasions, the socially anxious mind cannot. We're stuck in the off mode but with all the alerts and notifications turned on to hypersensitive. It feels a lot like being asked to give a speech to a crowd of people only your mouth is taped shut and all the fire alarms are going off.

The saddest part is that most of us are very creative individuals, meself excluded 'cause OMG what is this book even.

We try to be part of a world out there, but we seem to be stuck in the one inside our heads. And that one is not rainbows and lollipops. Not saying the real world is rainbows and lollipops, but at least the world offers the possibility to search those things out.

Dr. Hendricksen argues that Social Anxiety brings about a disruptive form of perfectionism in a person. People with S.A.D. believe that in order to escape judgment or to assuage the fear of 'being found out that we are inferior to others,' every social interaction must be absolutely perfect. And that can get in the way of building connections or relationships or even just our ability to live in the moment.

People have told me often that I am a perfectionist, or its less endearing sister term, a control freak. Why, yes. I believe that is true. But in my case it is a slightly different form of outright trying to control the world. Even though I try to control how people remember me or what they think of me, deep down I know the fact that I cannot control the world around me. I have learned to accept that. What I cannot seem to accept is that I seem incapable of rolling with the changes. As I understand it, I should be able to control at least myself. I should be able to control how my mind thinks, or how I respond to a situation, or what my body does or looks like. At the very least, I should be able to control myself. Otherwise, what's the point of doing anything? Nothing is ever going to be in your hands.

Help us learn how to let that go. Help us learn to let things go, period. The problem with fear and anxiety is how much you ruminate over something. Just mulling it in your head over and over and over until there is nothing left but self-loathing and dissatisfaction.

My brother jokes that I am a world champion in holding grudges. While he is not wrong, I am not sure he understands why I hold grudges at all. And part of the reason is I cannot let things go. Events, that one embarrassing time I did something stupid, or said something dumb. Or that one time someone called me out on something. I ruminate. And because I ruminate, I can't let go.

It's no secret that I have a hard time doing the simplest of things. I hold myself to the utmost of perfectionist standards. And yet if I mess up, or worse, if someone calls me out on messing up, all that agony and effort was for naught. And that makes me angry. I'm trying. I'm trying the hardest I can. Why can't people give me a break?

And I suppose that's what we want most of all, isn't it? Just someone to give us a break. We're trying aren't we? We're always trying.

I've always thought that is the most tragic part of living with Social Anxiety. There's no breathing room. You can't get away from society. People are everywhere. Pervasive. It's not like you can just back off from the world, turn it on mute, and just catch your breath. It's not like you should. And I've always been furious at people who do it. I can't catch a break for one second in my two and half decades of trying. What gives you the right?

But that's a different topic.

Perhaps that is why we learn to associate our cage with comfort. It's the closest we can get to being on our own, the closest we can get to getting a break.

That shouldn't have to be the case.

Our cage should not be our solace. I mean, it's a cage. What I'm asking you to do, what I'm begging you to do, all you friends and family and therapists out there, break us out of that cage. We may have the key, but we don't know where the lock is. Help us find it. Help us open the door.

And set us free.

Epilogue

I would sort of like to end with saying two things. Thank you. Thank you for going on this journey with me. Thank you for picking this up and deciding it was worth your time for a read. Thank you for giving me a chance and a voice to try to make a difference. And I hope it did, make a difference that is.

I hope it gave insight, I hope it gave some muddled form of clarity. And I hope it helped give people like me a voice when we feel we don't have one. Or can't have one. Or believe we shouldn't even have one.

I wish I was Dr. Hendricksen. I wish I could give you some tried and tested and research-proven tools to beat Social Anxiety. But all I can do is scream "Help us!" and try to explain what we mean when we say that. "Help us like this," and "Help us to do this instead of that." And maybe we need that. Just an on-the-ground perspective of what living with this, this petulant curse, feels like and what we need to beat it.

And I still say beat Social Anxiety. Even though I don't believe it will ever go away, I want to get to a point where I can at least pull my life back from its grubby paws whenever it shows itself again. That would be victory enough. And I want the same thing for all of us.

To beat that bastard into submission. It's our life. It's about time we figured out how to reclaim it.

The second thing I wanted to say was, I'm sorry.

I'm sorry for taking you on this journey. I'm sorry if it was triggering, or it made you feel angry or hopeless at times. I'm sorry I am not a better writer to make this easier on you. This is where you pay me a compliment and say "Oh no, hun; you're an excellent writer. Very passable."

The truth is, this was hard to write. It was hard to look at the darkest parts of me and try to put them into words to share. So I'm sorry if it came across as confusing at times. But it really was the best I could do. And I'm scared my best wasn't good enough. But I believe in the purpose I set out to fulfill. I have to believe in that.

If you're like me, then I'm sorry you felt the need to read this book. I'm sorry you're struggling with Social Anxiety.

No one else is going to say that to you.

Because chances are not a lot of people are going to understand. Not even most therapists.

So if you are a therapist who picked up this volume of drabbles, I wanted to say thank you. Thank you for trying. I hope psychoanalyzing me helped. And I hope it helps your patients.

That's my life in a nutshell, isn't it?

Thank you.

And I'm sorry.

And one of these days, I'm going to stop saying 'sorry.'

Here's to fighting for that day.

P.S.

When I started writing this, it was my last day of being 25, and I had woken up happy. I am now several months into being 26. And I have had to fight to maintain my 'happy.'

My weight has skyrocketed since then. I have stopped eating. And started eating. And stopped again. And so on.

My mood has dipped. And come back up.

I've had good days. I've had not so good days.

But I am still in the fight.

And I am finally done.

With this book I mean! Not with life. Life is fine. The book is done. Should have clarified. Oopsie.

When I started writing this, it was my last day of 25 and I was lost for what to do, guided only by the north star that is a sense of purpose of getting my thoughts out there. My north star to the turbulent sea that is my mind.

Today, though I am done, I feel just as scared as when I started writing. Because now comes the judgment. And we know well how I feel about that.

I stared at the email that had been waiting in the draft folder for weeks as I struggled to dredge up the nerve to hit send. I wanted so badly for this to be out in the world, in eager hands and more eager minds. But the looming threat of a hundred nos from a hundred editors and publishing houses before that one yes? That's a lot to ask of me.

I paced my bedroom, back and forth and back and forth and back and forth, determined to carve a rutt into the floor. Renn had long since grown bored of the monotonous entertainment and retired onto my pillow for a nap.

My feet hurt, heels sore, begging for reprieve.

I stopped. Cast a furtive glance at the laptop on the desk, the email still there, still haunting. Like a shadow in the corner that never seems to get enough light regardless of how many lights you turn on. A digital phantom.

I blew a sigh to the white-plastered ceiling, a frustrated prayer. The hundredth one I had blown in the past couple of hours, perhaps the trillionth in the past few weeks.

I had finished the draft ages ago. Read it. Reread it. Obsessed over it. Mucked it up, un-mucked it up.

There was no more stalling to do. The email sat ready, its precious cargo digitally clipped on like an express package about to be ripped open and devoured and torn to shreds and stitched back together. Like my heart was about to be.

I shuddered. Arms hugged my torso trying to find comfort in the face of impending trials.

"I can do this."

It wasn't a particularly creative mantra. And certainly not one that was readily believed in.

"I can do this."

I sat down in the chair, its wood now cold to the touch. I wondered if it had missed the warmth of a body or if it enjoyed being on its own.

No. Stop it. Distractions.

I reached to drag the cursor to the send button but it had been resting there for the past few weeks. I wonder if anyone had invented a program where digital cobwebs form on a cursor that has been static too long. It would be a very pointless program. But cool nonetheless.

I scratched my head, my newly dyed red hair bright in the sunlight from the window. Yeah, I dyed my hair red in an effort to work up the courage to send this stupid file. It's a whole coping thing.

Doesn't matter.

A deep breath, a snake-like strike. And the button on send had been pressed.

Your email is being sent.

The words danced on the screen. And then they didn't.

Before I had time to catch up, I realized I had reflexively hit *UNDO*. My brain finally arrived at the party with a "What the actual fuck, dude?"

Stupid.

This time I took a deep breath, held it, and dragged the cursor to the send button again. And hovered there.

My lungs began to burn for air. I felt the familiar tremble in my hands, the cursor gently vibrating on the screen.

In a forced rush of air, I hit send and leaped out of my chair. What followed can only be described as a manic raindance done by a drunk hooligan.

10. 9. 8.

Shit.

7. 6. 5.

Fuck.

4. 3. 2.

Oh my God.

1.

Bismillah.

Email sent.

It was done. I had done it. I had actually done it. The automated reply a second later scared the literal shit out of me. But I had done it.

Now we wait.

But something didn't feel right. How could this be an ending? It was really over?

I sat down again and opened the file I had just sent. Opened the last page. And left a last little message. For you.

*This has now seen the light of day. I succeeded.
Your turn.*